Severe Acute Respiratory Syndrome

From Benchtop to Bedside

Severe Acute Respiratory Syndrome

From Benchtop to Bedside

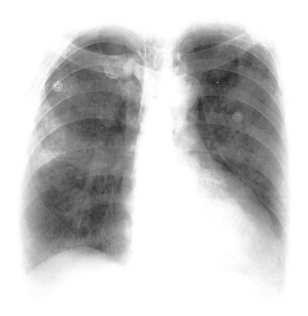

edited by

Joseph J Y Sung

The Chinese University of Hong Kong

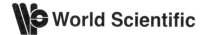

World Scientific

NEW JERSEY • LONDON • SINGAPORE • BEIJING • SHANGHAI • HONG KONG • TAIPEI • CHENNAI

Published by

World Scientific Publishing Co. Pte. Ltd.

5 Toh Tuck Link, Singapore 596224

USA office: Suite 202, 1060 Main Street, River Edge, NJ 07661

UK office: 57 Shelton Street, Covent Garden, London WC2H 9HE

British Library Cataloguing-in-Publication Data
A catalogue record for this book is available from the British Library.

SEVERE ACUTE RESPIRATORY SYNDROME
From Benchtop to Bedside

ISBN 981-238-753-6

Typeset by Stallion Press.

Printed in Singapore by World Scientific Printers (S) Pte Ltd

Contents

Contributors

AT Ahuja
Department of Diagnostic
  Radiology & Organ Imaging
Prince of Wales Hospital
The Chinese University of
  Hong Kong
Shatin, N.T.
Hong Kong

GE Antonio
Department of Diagnostic
  Radiology & Organ Imaging
Prince of Wales Hospital
The Chinese University of
  Hong Kong
Shatin, N.T.
Hong Kong

Paul KS Chan
Department of Microbiology
Prince of Wales Hospital
The Chinese University of
  Hong Kong
Shatin, New Territories
Hong Kong

Louis Y Chan
Hospital Authority
Hong Kong

Chen Wei Qing
School of Public Health
Sun Yat-sen University
Guangzhou, China

Gregory Cheng
Department of Medicine &
  Therapeutics
Prince of Wales Hospital
The Chinese University of
  Hong Kong
Shatin, N.T.
Hong Kong

Chi Ming Leung
Department of Psychiatry
Prince of Wales Hospital
The Chinese University of
  Hong Kong
Shatin, N.T.
Hong Kong

TF Fok
Department of Paediatrics
Prince of Wales Hospital
The Chinese University of
  Hong Kong
Shatin, N.T.
Hong Kong

Charles D Gomersall
Department of Anaesthesia and
  Intensive Care
Prince of Wales Hospital
The Chinese University of
  Hong Kong
Shatin, N.T.
Hong Kong

Hong Fung
Hospital Authority
Hong Kong

David SC Hui
Department of Medicine and
  Therapeutics
Prince of Wales Hospital
Chinese University of Hong Kong
Shatin, New Territories
Hong Kong

Gavin M Joynt
Department of Anaesthesia and
  Intensive Care
Prince of Wales Hospital
The Chinese University of
  Hong Kong
Shatin, N.T.
Hong Kong

Irene Kam
Department of Psychiatry
Prince of Wales Hospital
The Chinese University of
  Hong Kong
Shatin, N.T.
Hong Kong

Timothy Kwok
Department of Geriatrics
Prince of Wales Hospital
The Chinese University of
  Hong Kong
Shatin, N.T.
Hong Kong

Nelson Lee
Department of Medicine &
  Therapeutics
Prince of Wales Hospital
The Chinese University of
  Hong Kong
Shatin, New Territories
Hong Kong

Sing Lee
Department of Psychiatry
Prince of Wales Hospital
The Chinese University of
  Hong Kong
Shatin, N.T.
Hong Kong

PC Leung
Department of Orthopaedics
Prince of Wales Hospital
The Chinese University of
  Hong Kong
Shatin, N.T.
Hong Kong

WK Leung
Department of Medicine &
  Therapeutics
Prince of Wales Hospital
The Chinese Univeristy of
  Hong Kong
Shatin, New Territories,
Hong Kong

SF Liu
Department of Medicine and
  Therapeutics
Prince of Wales Hospital
The Chinese University of
  Hong Kong
Shatin, N.T.
Hong Kong

YM Dennis Lo
Department of Chemical
  Pathology
Center for Emerging Infectious
  Diseases
The Chinese University of
  Hong Kong
Shatin, N.T.
Hong Kong

Violeta Lopez
The Nethersole School
  of Nursing
The Chinese University of
  Hong Kong
Shatin, N.T.
Hong Kong

Donald Lyon
Surrey and Sussex Healthcare
  NHS Trust
United Kingdom

Enders KO Ng
Department of Chemical Pathology
Prince of Wales Hospital
The Chinese University of
  Hong Kong
Shatin, New Territories
Hong Kong

Timothy H Rainer
Accident and Emergency Medicine
  Academic Unit
Prince of Wales Hospital
The Chinese University of
  Hong Kong
Shatin, N.T.
Hong Kong

Joseph JY Sung
Department of Medicine &
  Therapeutics
Center for Emerging Infectious
  Diseases
The Chinese University of
  Hong Kong
Shatin, N.T.
Hong Kong

David R Thompson
The Nethersole School
  of Nursing
The Chinese University of
  Hong Kong
Shatin, N.T.
Hong Kong

Peter Tong
Department of Medicine and
  Therapeutics
Prince of Wales Hospital
The Chinese University of
  Hong Kong
Shatin, N.T.
Hong Kong

KT Wong
Department of Diagnostic
  Radiology & Organ Imaging
Prince of Wales Hospital
The Chinese University of
  Hong Kong
Shatin, N.T.
Hong Kong

Raymond SM Wong
Department of Haematology &
  Haematological Oncology
Prince of Wales Hospital
The Chinese University of
  Hong Kong
Shatin, N.T.
Hong Kong

Wong Tze Wai
Department of Community and
  Family Medicine
Prince of Wales Hospital
The Chinese University of
  Hong Kong
Shatin, N.T.
Hong Kong

Vincent Wong
Department of Medicine and
  Therapeutics
The Prince of Wales Hospital
The Chinese University of
  Hong Kong
Shatin, N.T.
Hong Kong

AKL Wu
Department of Medicine &
  Therapeutics
Prince of Wales Hospital
The Chinese University of
  Hong Kong
Shatin, N.T.
Hong Kong

Yun Kwok Wing
Department of Psychiatry
Prince of Wales Hospital
The Chinese University of
  Hong Kong
Shatin, N.T.
Hong Kong

1

A Global Outbreak

Joseph JY Sung

SARS is the first severe and readily transmissible disease that emerged in the 21st century. SARS has a unique capacity of spreading quickly in hospitals and clinics, affecting thousands of healthcare workers in a very short time. The booming international air travel in recent decades has also enabled the infection to be quickly spread across the continents and becoming an international threat. One infected tourist from China checked into a hotel in Hong Kong and spread the infection to three countries. As at 3 July 2003, 32 countries have been affected and 8439 patients infected around the world.[1] On 12 March, the World Health Organization (WHO) issued the First Global Alert against an atypical pneumonia of unknown cause not responding to antibiotics. Three days later on 15 March, WHO issued the Second Global Alert in which, for the first time this new disease was named Severe Acute Respiratory Syndrome with its case definition laid down. Because of the seriousness of the infection and the high infectivity, "WHO regards every country with an international airport, or bordering an area having a recent local transmission, as at potential risk of an outbreak."[2] Travel advisory was issued based on (1) the magnitude of the outbreak in those countries;

(2) the pattern of local transmission; and (3) exportation of probable cases to other countries. Guidance was provided to the general public to postpone non-essential travel to areas with local transmissions and that met the above criteria. These travel advisories have generated huge and unprecedented economic and social impacts in countries like China (including Hong Kong SAR), Canada, Singapore and Taiwan.

The following is an account of events that happened within three weeks from late February to mid-March.

WHERE DID IT FIRST START?

The first cases of SARS are now known to have emerged in mid-November 2002 in Guangdong province of southern China. On November 27, the Global Public Health Intelligence Network (GPHIN), a computer application developed by the Heath Canada and used by WHO, picked up emails reporting atypical pneumonia in Foshan city of Guangdong. GPHIN is a customized search engine that continuously scans world Internet communications for rumors and reports of suspicious disease events in over 950 news feeds and electronic discussion groups around the world. Two months later, WHO received emails regarding atypical pneumonia outbreaks in Guangdong province. This was subsequently confirmed officially by the Ministry of Health of China as an outbreak of acute respiratory syndrome that involved 305 patients and five deaths in Guangdong. Around 30% of the cases affected were healthcare workers in the hospitals. WHO was further informed that the outbreak which involved six municipalities was not influenza. Further investigation from laboratories in China ruled out anthrax, pulmonary plague, leptospirosis and hemorrhagic fever. In the meantime, the disease was carried outside the country by travelers.

HOTEL M

Evidence has shown that during the period from late February to early March, there was a cluster of infected patients from southern China who traveled to Hong Kong. The most prominent case was a Professor of Nephrology, who had treated patients in his home town, and who came to Hong Kong on 21 February 2003 to attend a wedding banquet of his relative.[3] He brought the virus to the ninth floor of a four-star hotel

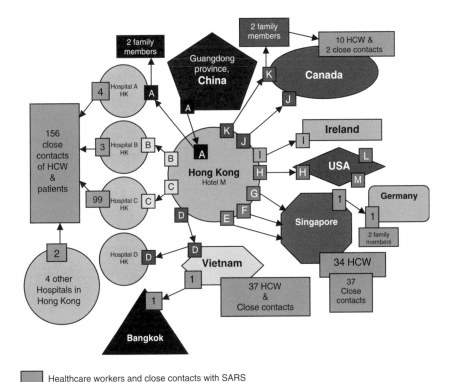

Fig. 1 Chain of transmission among guests at Hotel M of Hong Kong, February–March 2003 (adopted from *MMWR* of CDC with permission).

(Hotel M) in Hong Kong (Fig. 1). This medical doctor infected at least 12 other guests and visitors on the 9th floor of the hotel. Days later, guests and visitors to the hotel seeded outbreaks in eight countries including Ireland, Vietnam, Singapore, Hong Kong and Toronto.

HANOI

On 28 February, a 48-year-old Chinese-American businessman was admitted to the French Hospital in Hanoi with a 3-day history of respiratory symptoms of pneumonia. He had previously been in Hong Kong, where he visited an acquaintance staying on the 9th floor of Hotel M. Dr. Carlo Urbani, an epidemiologist from the WHO office in Hanoi, examined this gentleman who had features of atypical pneumonia. On 5 March, the businessman was air transferred to the Princess Margaret

Hospital in Hong Kong. Seven healthcare workers in Hanoi who had cared for him became ill. WHO staff were sent to Vietnam to help manage the epidemic. By 11 March, at least 20 hospital workers in Hanoi's French Hospital came down with the same symptoms. Dr. Urbani notified the WHO Regional Office for the Western Pacific. The WHO headquarters move into a heightened state of alert. Dr. Urbani continued to treat cases at the Hanoi French Hospital. On 11 March, Dr. Urbani was invited to give a presentation on tropical diseases in Bangkok. He was ill upon arrival and was immediately hospitalized. Dr. Urbani died of respiratory failure on 29 March in a Bangkok hospital.

SINGAPORE

On 1 March, a 26-year-old former flight attendant was admitted to a hospital in Singapore with respiratory symptoms. This patient was also a guest on the 9th floor of Hotel M in Hong Kong. The government of Singapore notified WHO on 15 March by urgent communication that a similar illness had been found in a 32-year-old physician who had treated cases with a severe respiratory symptom in Singapore, all subsequently linked to Hotel M. The Singapore physician traveled to the United States for a medical conference and at the end of the conference boarded a return flight from New York. The physician and his two accompanying family members were removed from the flight at a stopover in Frankfurt where the three were immediately isolated and placed under hospital care.

HONG KONG

On 28 February, a 26-year-old man presented to the Prince of Wales Hospital with a 3-day history of fever, chills and rigor. He was diagnosed to have upper respiratory tract infection and discharged at the hospital's emergency room. His fever did not respond to the medication and the patient returned on 4 March with productive cough. During that visit, he also had diarrhea with brownish loose stool and vomited undigested food. He denied any history of travel (until after the story of Hotel M was disclosed in Hong Kong). Chest examination showed a bronchial breath sound at the right upper zone. Chest X-ray showed a right upper lobe consolidation. A diagnosis of community-acquired pneumonia was made and he was admitted to ward 8A. From March 6 to March 14, because of his shortness of breath, this patient was treated with bronchodilator via a jet nebulizer delivered by oxygen for a total of seven days. Within two weeks, a total of 156 patients were hospitalized, of whom 138 were identified as either secondary cases or tertiary cases of this index case. This included 69 healthcare workers (20 doctors, 34 nurses, 15 allied health workers); 16 medical students who had worked in the index ward; and 54 patients who were either nursed in the same medical ward or had visited their relatives.

TORONTO

A 78-year-old Toronto woman who had been a guest on the 9th floor of Hotel M developed fever, myalgia, sore throat and progressive dyspnea two days after she returned home. She died at home on March 5. Several family members of the index patient subsequently developed symptoms of pneumonia and was admitted to Scarborough Grace Hospital, which became the epicenter of the infection. SARS spread to healthcare workers and other patients in the hospital prior to a significant awareness of the disease in the local medical community. Other Toronto hospitals were involved when patients were transferred between institutions. This led to additional patients, healthcare workers and visitors contracting the disease in hospitals in the Toronto area. On March 14, WHO was alerted by Health Canada that steps had been taken to alert hospital workers, ambulance services and public health units across the provinces of the country.

BEIJING

On March 15, a 72-year-old man boarded a flight from Hong Kong to Beijing. He visited ward 8A at the Prince of Wales Hospital from 4 to 9 March and developed a fever on 11 March. On this flight, there were at least 22 passengers who were subsequently confirmed to have SARS, including travelers from Taiwan, Singapore, Bangkok, Hong Kong and Inner Mongolia. This patient died of the disease in Beijing. In late March, the Chinese authorities issued updated data on cases and deaths relating to outbreak of atypical pneumonia in Guangdong province reported earlier, raising the cumulative total number of cases from 305 to 792, and of death from 5 to 31. On 4 April, a retired medical doctor in Beijing wrote to television channels in China exposing an epidemic of SARS in the city. He was then interviewed by *TIME* magazine and disclosed a cover-up of the epidemic. On 20 April, the health authority reported the number of SARS cases in Beijing which jumped from dozens to 346.

GLOBAL EPIDEMIC AND INTERNATIONAL RESPONSE

From November 2002 to 3 July 2003, the day when the last SARS cases were reported to the WHO, there was a total of 8439 cases reported from 32 countries involving six continents. The last case in this epidemic was reported from Toronto, Canada on 27 June 2003. Eight hundred and twelve people died, making an overall mortality of 9.6%. There is a wide variation in mortality among the heavily hit countries, ranging from 6.5% to 16.9%.

In combating of the serious infection, the international scientific community has come to put their efforts together.

On 15 March 2003, the day WHO issued an emergency travel advisory in response to SARS, it set up a network of scientists from 11 laboratories around the world to expedite the identification of the causative agent of SARS. They were asked to share among themselves scientific data and clinical specimens. The collaboration was continued through daily teleconferences and use of the WHO website to post electron microscopy pictures of candidate viruses, protocols for testing, phylogenetic trees, PCR primer sequences and results of various diagnostic tests. These arrangements allow simultaneous analyses of samples from the same patients in several laboratories with different approaches. With these efforts, in just about one month, a new species of coronavirus now called SARS-CoV was identified. The clinical management groups from different countries were also connected by teleconferences to share experiences in the clinical management of SARS patients. Information, including natural course of the disease, incubation period, clinical presentation and response to various modalities of treatment, was discussed. It is through these international collaborative efforts of unprecedented scale that our knowledge of the disease and hence its management scheme can be developed in such a short time.

With the exception of AIDS, most new diseases that emerged in the past two decades have features that limit their capacity to pose a major

Table 1 Cumulative Number of Reported Probable Cases of SARS from
1 Nov 2002 to 3 July 2003

Country	Cumulative No. of Cases	No. of Death	No. Recovered	Date Last Probable Case Reported
Australia	5	0	5	12 May 2003
Brazil	1	0	1	9 June 2003
Canada	251	38	193	27 June 2003
China	5327	348	4933	25 June 2003
Hong Kong SAR	1755	298	1429	11 June 2003
Macao SAR	1	0	1	21 May 2003
Taiwan	674	84	498	19 June 2003
Colombia	1	0	1	5 May 2003
Finland	1	0	1	7 May 2003
France	7	0	6	9 May 2003
Germany	10	0	9	4 June 2003
India	3	0	3	13 May 2003
Indonesia	2	0	2	23 April 2003
Italy	4	0	4	29 April 2003
Kuwait	1	0	1	9 April 2003
Malaysia	5	2	3	20 May 2003
Mongolia	9	0	9	6 May 2003
New Zealand	1	0	1	30 April 2003
Philippines	14	2	12	15 May 2003
Republic of Ireland	1	0	1	21 March 2003
Republic of Korea	3	0	3	14 May 2003
Romania	1	0	1	27 March 2003
Russian Federation	1	0	0	31 May 2003
Singapore	206	32	171	18 May 2003
South Africa	1	1	0	9 April 2003
Spain	1	0	1	2 April 2003
Sweden	3	0	3	18 April 2003
Switzerland	1	0	1	17 March 2003
Thailand	9	2	7	7 June 2003
United Kingdom	4	0	4	29 April 2003
United States	73	0	65	23 June 2003
Vietnam	63	5	58	14 April 2003
TOTAL	8439	812	7427	

threat to international public health. Avian influenza, Nipah virus, Ebola virus, and Hanta virus did not establish efficient human-to-human transmission. Others require a vector for the transmission. SARS is unusual in its high morbidity and mortality. Indeed, the endemic in early 2003 mimics the 1918 influenza panendmic. SARS-CoV shared several biological features with influenza A virus. Both viruses are zoonoses. Both have dual tissue tropism for respiratory and gastrointestinal tissues. As RNA viruses, both possess mechanisms for mutations and generate genetic variability. At the turn of 20th century, it took three panendemics before influenza was brought under control. Considering the rapidity of spread of SARS and the high mortality of this disease in such a short time, this formidable disease has more serious effects compared to influenza.

The SARS endemics have exposed problems of the healthcare system of many countries. Weaknesses of the public health system, fragmentation of organization of national healthcare, slow communication and inadequate alert system are some of the lessons learned by the international community. The final success in the containment of the disease was the result of efforts from high-level governmental intervention. Legislation of prevention and control of infectious disease and promotion of public alertness and response turned out to be the crucial factors in controlling SARS. Although the recent endemic appeared to be contained, the world should not be complacent. There are still many unanswered questions about SARS-CoV and the disease it causes. Scientists and clinicians around the world should continue their joint efforts until we have a thorough understanding of the nature of the virus, its source, mode of transmission, pathological effects and therapeutic options. Until then, the world is still under the shadow of the come back of SARS.

2

The Epidemiology of SARS

Wong Tze Wai, Chen Wei-Qing

INTRODUCTION

In late 2002, a novel clinical entity manifesting as a febrile upper respiratory illness, progressing in some patients to a life-threatening pneumonia, emerged in Guangdong province in southern China. It attracted international attention through an explosive outbreak in Hong Kong, and was subsequently defined as severe acute respiratory syndrome (SARS) in March 2003.[1] It quickly spread to 25 provinces/cities in China and to 32 countries/regions around the world. From 16 November 2002 to 5 July 2003 (when World Health Organization (WHO) announced that all known person-to-person transmission of SARS had ceased), a total of 8437 probable SARS cases were reported to the WHO from 32 countries/ regions; with a total of 813 deaths and a case fatality rate of 9.6%.[2] A total of 5327 probable SARS cases with 348 deaths were diagnosed in mainland China, according to the WHO criteria.[2]

The first known case of SARS was reported in Foshan (a city in Guangdong province) on 16 November 2002. Three family members of the index case were also affected. Subsequently, small clusters of patients

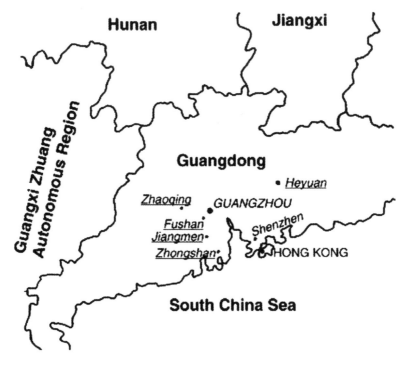

Fig. 1 Location of cities in which SARS cases occurred in Guangdong province, southern China. The cities involved in the early phase of the outbreak are underlined.

with SARS were noted in Heyuan, Zhongshan, Jiangmen, Shengzhen and Zhaoqing (Fig. 1) from November 2002 to January 2003. Following the transfer of a patient from Zhongshan, a major cluster of cases occurred in Guangzhou leading subsequently to the global alert.[3]

The spread of SARS outside Guangdong province occurred when a nephrologist from Guangzhou traveled to Hong Kong on 21 February 2003. He had a 5-day history of respiratory symptoms and was admitted to a hospital on the second day of his stay in Hong Kong. While staying in a hotel in Hong Kong, he was believed to have infected a couple from Toronto, Canada; a businessman who later traveled to Hanoi, Vietnam; three tourists from Singapore; and a number of Hong Kong residents. These victims, in their turn, started large outbreaks in their destinations.[1,4] On 1 March 2003, a general hospital in Beijing admitted the first SARS patient from Shanxi, who was infected while doing business in Guangzhou. In this hospital, he transmitted the disease to healthcare workers (HCWs) who attended to him without adequate personal protection. Then, SARS began to spread in Beijing. Subsequently, suspected SARS patients, mostly imported from infected areas, were reported in other regions of the mainland.

AGENT, HOST AND ENVIRONMENT

Agent

The etiological link of a coronavirus with the SARS epidemic, now termed SARS-associated coronavirus (SARS-CoV) was first established in Hong Kong,[5] and it was quickly confirmed by collaborative studies in various institutions throughout the world.[6,7] The characteristic features of SARS-CoV are covered in Chapter 3.

Host

To date, human is the only confirmed host of SARS, and the SARS patient is the direct or indirect source of infection of others. There is no evidence of the existence of a sub-clinical carrier state.

SARS patients

Clinical SARS patients pose a significant health risk to household contacts and HCWs. Isolates of SARS-CoV were found from the nasopharyngeal aspirates and an open lung biopsy of two SARS patients.[5,6] Droplets and aerosols of varying sizes can be generated by coughing, sneezing or even talking, and disease transmission by large droplets is currently considered as the most important route. Certain treatment procedures (e.g., non-invasive ventilation, endotracheal intubation, open tracheal suction, and bronchoscopy) may further enhance the risk of infection. The use of nebulizers has been incriminated in a hospital outbreak in Hong Kong.[8,9] However, this has not been supported by epidemiological evidence.[10] A study of SARS patients in Guangzhou showed that IgM antibody titres to the SARS-CoV peaked during the acute or early convalescent phase (week 3) of their illnesses and declined by the end of week 12, while IgG peaked at week 12.[11] Although it is still unclear at what stage of the disease virus shedding occurs,[12] the viral load in the nasopharyngeal aspirates of patients in a community outbreak peaked at 10 days after the onset of symptoms.[13]

Superspreaders

The occurrence of a large number of cases that originated from a single patient has led to the description of "superspreaders," or more appropriately, "superspreading events."[14] The patient (a visitor from Guangzhou) who was responsible for the epidemic in Hong Kong, Vietnam, Canada and Singapore, infected at least 10 guests staying in the same hotel.[15] The index patient in a major hospital outbreak in Hong Kong infected more than 40 HCWs in the ward where he stayed.[10] In Singapore, five patients were responsible for a total of 170 suspected and probable cases of SARS.[14] These "superspreaders" have been described in other viral infections, such as Ebola hemorrhagic fever,[16] rubella[17] and hemolytic streptococcal infection.[18] It is important to study whether host factors, different strains of the virus and/or the characteristic environmental factors are responsible for the "superspreading event." Besides environmental and agent factors, further studies on the infectivity of the SARS patient throughout the course of the illness and possible routes of disease transmission would shed light on this phenomenon. One other important factor for the "superspreading event" is the inadequate infection-control measures taken by HCWs, especially at the early phase of the epidemic, which has facilitated disease transmission.

Asymptomatic carriers

An important question is whether an asymptomatic human carrier of SARS-CoV exists, and if it does, the duration of this state. In a serological study of over 100 family contacts of SARS patients and over 800 medical students in the Chinese University of Hong Kong, no evidence of infection was detected (Wong R, *et al.* unpublished data). Except for the common source outbreak in Amoy Gardens in Hong Kong, a positive history of contact with a known SARS patient can be obtained in most SARS cases. This fact and the absence of seropositive family contacts, strongly suggest the absence of asymptomatic carriers. If asymptomatic carriers do exist, public health control and eradication of the SARS will be extremely difficult.

Animal reservoir

The identification of a non-human reservoir of infection and the extent of the prevalence of the virus in this reservoir are of epidemiological importance not only in tracing the origin of this mysterious epidemic, but also in the prevention of a future outbreak. There is evidence that SARS might have originated from wild animals. In a recent collaborative study in Hong Kong and Shenzhen, researchers isolated several coronaviruses that were genetically closely related to the SARS-CoV from 6 masked palm civets (*Paguma larvata*) and a raccoon-dog (*Nyctereutes procyonoides*). They also detected antibodies against the SARS-CoV in a Chinese ferret badger (*Melogale moschata*) in a market in Shenzhen in the southern Chinese province of Guangdong.[19] Comparison between the complete genomic sequence of the SARS-CoV published in May and the strains of coronaviruses sampled from the wild animals, indicated that 99.8% of nucleotides in the gene are the same and that the SARS-CoV lacks 29 nucleotides in the gene for a protein of unknown function, which is attached to the inside of the virus's protective coat. In contrast, an investigation by researchers at the Chinese Agricultural University in Beijing failed to identify SARS-like coronaviruses in 732 animals from 54 wild and 11 domesticated species in southern China, including the palm civets.[20] Uncertainties still remain over the exact source of the SARS-CoV, and the role of wildlife in the SARS epidemic is being evaluated by the WHO. In a recent paper Ng (2003) postulated that roof rats might play a part in the transmission of SARS in a large-scale community outbreak in Amoy Gardens in Hong Kong. One major weakness of his hypothesis is the abrupt decline of the outbreak, an unlikely observation given the high infestation of rats and the difficulties of eradicating them. Another piece of evidence against the hypothesis is that, to date, infection of laboratory rats has not been successful. The macaque monkey (*Macaca fascicularis*) is the only laboratory animal model reported thus far.[22]

The Environment

The hospital is a high-risk environment for the spread of SARS. Many SARS outbreaks originated from hospitals where SARS patients were treated.[15,23] In the first major hospital outbreak in Hong Kong, epidemiological data and ventilation study results suggested that, besides droplet spread, airborne transmission might play a role through faulty ventilation of the hospital ward.[10] Besides the hospital, some large community outbreaks have also been attributed to environmental factors. In Amoy Gardens, a private housing estate in Hong Kong, a common source outbreak occurred in March 2003.[24] Virus-laden fecal discharge by an index patient was believed to have created infectious aerosols within the sewer system. Aerosols could then enter the bathrooms of the residents in the same building from the sewage pipe (through dried air traps on the bathroom floor) by the suction effect of the bathroom exhaust fan. The aerosols were believed to have been disseminated to households in the higher floors by a "plume effect" in the re-entrant (the space exterior to the bathroom, between two adjacent apartment blocks). There is supporting evidence of an airborne spread of the aerosols from the re-entrant in this building to other buildings (Li, *et al.*, unpublished data). The hypothesis of infected roof rats in the environment lacks supportive serological evidence.[21]

Routes of Disease Transmission

Transmission through droplets

The primary mode of transmission of SARS is believed to be by droplet spread through close person-to-person contact.[14] Most cases of SARS have involved people who cared for or lived with, or had direct contact with infectious materials (such as respiratory secretions) from a SARS patient. The occurrence of clusters of cases among HCWs caring for, and family members of, SARS patients strongly suggested that transmission of SARS occurs primarily by contact with large respiratory droplets in the close vicinity of an infected person. In an experimental study, SARS-CoV were recovered from the nose and throat of two macaques inoculated with the virus.[22]

Transmission through contact with fomites

Recent data have indicated that the virus may remain viable for considerable periods on a dry surface (up to 24 hours).[2] Hence, touching surfaces or objects that are contaminated with SARS-CoV may introduce the latter into the mucus membranes of the eye, nose or possibly, the mouth. Virus spread via fomites is also compatible with the observed higher risk of infection among HCWs and family contacts of SARS patients.

Transmission through the fecal-oral route

SARS-CoV has been detected in the feces of patients by RT-PCR and viral culture.[13] The virus is stable in feces (and urine) at room temperature for at least 1 to 2 days and up to 4 days in stools from patients with diarrhea (which has a higher pH than normal stool).[25] A significant proportion of SARS patients in the outbreak in Guangzhou, the Amoy Gardens outbreak in Hong Kong, and the hospital outbreaks in Hong Kong and Canada presented with diarrhea.[1,3,4,13] Hence, despite the lack of definitive epidemiological evidence, it is possible that SARS-CoV may be transmitted through the fecal-oral route.

Transmission through airborne spread

There is some evidence that airborne transmission may have a role in some settings, such as the community outbreak at Amoy Gardens in Hong Kong that occurred in late March to early April 2003, affecting over 300 patients. The source was attributed to a SARS patient who had diarrhea, and the disease was believed to have spread to residents in other flats by virus-laden aerosols that somehow traveled from the sewer to the "re-entrant" outside the bathroom (either through a leaking sewage drain, or via the dried-up air trap of the floor drain in the bathroom). The infectious aerosols might have dispersed upwards as a rising plume to other flats.[24] Certain medical procedures, like endotracheal intubation, open tracheal suction and nasopharyngeal aspiration might produce aerosols that facilitate disease transmission. Whether inadequate ventilation in a crowded hospital environment has contributed to the hospital outbreak requires further investigation.

THE SARS EPIDEMIC: A SUMMARY OF EPIDEMIOLOGICAL CHARACTERISTICS

1. *In most countries affected by SARS, the epidemic started as hospital outbreaks with a high rate of infection among HCWs at the early stage, when there was inadequate personal protective equipment or when infection control procedures had not been vigorously implemented.*

Towards the end of February 2003, SARS was introduced from Guangdong province in southern China to Hong Kong, which as a major transport hub, exported the disease to other cities in China and beyond. Hanoi, Singapore, and Toronto were first affected, followed by Beijing and Taipei. In these cities, the outbreaks became the initial "hot zones" of SARS, affecting a large number of HCWs and their family contacts, as well as other patients in the hospital and their visitors. The high attack rate amongst hospital staff is a constant feature in the outbreaks in all these cities. From the hospitals, the disease then spread to the community, where community transmission then prevailed. After the hospital outbreak, community spread began in the district where the hospital was situated.

One of the biggest concerns in the spread of SARS has been the high rate of infections amongst HCW and in healthcare settings. In the Greater Toronto area, 111 of 144 SARS cases had an exposure history to SARS in a hospital, and 73 (51%) were HCWs.[26] In Hong Kong, among 138 cases of secondary and tertiary spread, 85 (62%) involved HCWs.[1] Most of these events occurred prior to the recognition of the disease, when infection-control precautions were inadequate.

2. While clustering of cases was typical in hospital outbreaks, sporadic cases occurred concurrently in the community.

The short incubation period (2 to 10 days with mean 5 days) of SARS and its ability to spread by respiratory droplets and fomites facilitated the clustering of cases, mostly HCWs in a hospital setting. Towards the later stage of the epidemic in China, most of the SARS cases were sporadic, with no definite history of exposure to an infectious source. Almost 50% to 60% of the SARS patients in Beijing and Guangzhou could not be traced to a known source. This might be explained by casual contact with a SARS patient who was not a family/close contact. Sporadic cases arising from contact with infectious materials in the environment have yet to be documented.

3. Rapid dissemination to major cities and local transmission in densely populated areas.

In the southern Chinese province of Guangdong, where the epidemic originated, SARS initially appeared as a small cluster of cases in the rural areas. The antecedent leading to the global alert was a major outbreak among HCWs in three hospitals in Guangzhou. This outbreak was traced to a "superspreader" (or more aptly, a superspreading event) who was transferred from Zhongshan county to one of the three hospitals for better quality medical care. This major outbreak then spread beyond the province to other countries through railway and air travel (described in Introduction).

Although probable SARS cases have been reported in 32 countries/regions in the world, local spread occurred in only seven countries/regions, all with high population density. In the other countries/regions, all the cases were imported.

4. *Herd immunity is very low in all the affected countries; the decline of the epidemic resulted from vigorous and effective public health measures.*

Tests on sera obtained before the SARS outbreak did not detect any specific antibodies against SARS-CoV, suggesting that almost everybody is susceptible to SARS. According to the classical SIR model in infectious disease epidemiology, the epidemic should only ebb when the herd immunity rises to a sufficiently high level, when the immune population offers protection against effective contact between the infectious and the susceptible groups. The basic reproductive rate, R_0, measures the infectiousness of a disease and corresponds to the average number of secondary cases generated by one primary case in a susceptible population. R_0 for SARS has been estimated to range from 2–4.[27] Various public health measures have been implemented, including prompt identification and isolation of cases, quarantine of contacts, public health educations on personal hygiene, the prevalent practice of using face-masks in public places, restriction of hospital visitors, travel restrictions, and temperature checks at airport and railway stations. The prompt identification and isolation of cases is probably the most important public health measure for controling the spread of the disease, while the value of quarantine measures has not been scientifically evaluated. (Vietnam was the first country declared SARS-free. Yet, the epidemic was largely limited to the hospitals, and no quarantine measures were implemented.) Singapore used the military to assist in contact tracing and enforcement of home quarantine. Through this and other measures (including screening of passengers at airports and seaports, concentration of SARS patients in a designated hospital, imposition of a no-visitors rule for all public hospitals, and use of a dedicated private ambulance service to transport all suspected cases) Singapore has successfully controled the SARS epidemic, and reported its last case on 11 May, 2003. About one month after the start of the outbreak in Hong Kong, quarantine measures were implemented. With intensified contact tracing and other public health measures, a substantial decline was observed and the epidemic ended by the end of June.

5. *Seasonality: SARS started in winter/spring and ended in summer.*

Like influenza, SARS exhibited a seasonal pattern. The disease first occurred in the winter of 2002. There were two waves in the global - epidemic. The first wave was from December 2002 to April 2003 in Guangdong, and the second wave from March 2003 to May 2003 in Beijing, Hong Kong, Singapore, Taiwan, and Toronto. Whether the observed seasonal pattern signifies another epidemic in winter is still uncertain.

6. *Risk factors for SARS among HCWs.*

Three major reasons for the spread of the infection to HCWs were: failure to apply isolation precautions to cases not yet identified as SARS; breaches of procedures; and inadequate precautions.[28] However, if every patient (including those without typical symptoms of SARS) is managed as if he/she is a potential case of SARS, this would have major implications for healthcare delivery. Another reason for the spread of SARS among HCWs was that infected workers continued to work at the early stage of their illness, spreading the disease to their colleagues and other patients. Early isolation of HCW with SARS is therefore essential, so as to minimize the risk to other co-workers. Adequate personal protective equipment is required in their daily work, in particular, when certain high-risk procedures are performed which might generate infectious droplets in the environment. These included nasopharyngeal aspiration, bronchoscopy, endotracheal intubation, airway suction, cardiopulmonary resuscitation, and possibly, the use of nebulizers and non-invasive ventilation procedures. In addition, nursing, feeding and cleaning the patients and their bedding also increase the risk of infection.

REFERENCES

1. Lee N, Hui D, Wu A, *et al.* A major outbreak of severe acute respiratory syndrome in Hong Kong. *N Engl J Med* 2003; **348**:1986–1994.

2. WHO a. Cumulative number of reported probable cases of SARS. Published online, 11 July 2003. http://www.who.int/csr/sars/country/2003_07_11/en/print.html.

3. Zhao Z, Zhang F, Xu M, *et al*. Description and clinical treatment of an early outbreak of severe acute respiratory syndrome (SARS) in Guangzhou, PR China. *J Med Microbiol* 2003;**52**:715–720.

4. Poutanen SM, Low DE, Henry B, *et al*. Identification of severe acute respiratory syndrome in Canada. *N Engl J Med* 2003;**348**: 1995–2005.

5. Peiris JSM, Lai ST, Poon LLM, *et al*. Coronavirus as a possible cause of severe acute respiratory syndrome. *Lancet* 2003a;**361**: 1319–1325.

6. Drosten C, Günther S, Preiser W, *et al*. Identification of a novel coronavirus in patients with severe acute respiratory syndrome. *N Engl J Med* 2003;**348**:1967–1976.

7. Ksiazek TG, Erdman D, Goldsmith CS, *et al*. A novel coronavirus associated with severe acute respiratory syndrome. SARS Working Group. *N Engl J Med* 2003;**348**:1953–1966.

8. Chan-Yeung M, Seto WH, Sung JY. Severe acute respiratory syndrome. *BMJ* 2003;**326**:1393.

9. Tomlinson B and Cockram C. SARS: Experience at Prince of Wales Hospital, Hong Kong. *Lancet* 2003;**361**:1486–1487.

10. Wong TW, Lee CK, Tam W, *et al*. Cluster of SARS among medical students exposed to single patient, Hong Kong. *Emerg Infecti Dis* 2004;**10**:269–275.

11. Li G, Chen X, Xu A. Profile of specific antibodies to the SARS-associated Coronavirus. *N England J Med* 2003;**349**(5):508–509.

12. Sampathkumar P, Temesgen Z, Smith TF, Thompson RL. SARS: Epidemiology, clinical presentation, management, and infection control measures. *Mayo Clin Proc* 2003;**78**:882–890.

13. Peiris JSM, Chu CM, Cheng VCC, *et al*. Clinical progression and viral load in a community outbreak of corona-associated SARS pneumonia: A prospective study. *Lancet* 2003b; published on-line May 9, 2003. http://image.thelancet.com/extras/03art4432web.pdf.

14. MMWR a. Severe acute respiratory syndrome — Singapore, 2003. *MMWR* 2003;**52**(18):405–411.

15. MMWR b. Update: Outbreak of severe acute respiratory syndrome — worldwide, 2003. *MMWR* 2003;**52**(12):241–248.

16. Khan AS, Tshioko FK, Heymann DL, *et al.* The resurgence of Ebola hemorrhagic fever, Democratic Republic of the Congo, 1995. *J Infect Dis* 1999;**179**(Suppl 1):S76–86.

17. Hattis RP, Halstead SB, Hermann KL, Witte JJ. Rubella in an immunized island population. *JAMA* 1973;**223**:1010–1021.

18. Hamburger M Jr, Green MJ, Hamburger VG. The problem of the "dangerous carrier" of hemolytic streptococci. II. Spread of infection by individuals with strongly positive nose cultures who expelled large numbers of hemolytic streptococci. *J Infect Dis* 1945;**77**:96–108.

19. Cyranoski D, Abbott A. Virus detectives seek source of SARS in China's wild animals. *Nature* 2003;**423**:467.

20. Clarke T. SARS: What have we learned? *Nature* 2003;**424**:121–126.

21. Ng SKC. Possible role of an animal vector in the SARS outbreak at Amoy Garden. *Lancet* 2003;**362**:570–572.

22. Fouchier RA, Kuiken T, Schutten M, *et al.* Aetiology: Koch's postulates fulfilled for SARS virus. *Nature* 2003;**423**:240.

23. Varia M, Wilson S, Sarwal S, *et al.* Investigation of a nosocomial outbreak of severe acute respiratory syndrome (SARS) in Toronto, Canada. *CMAJ* 2003;**169**(4):285–292.

24. Department of Health, Hong Kong Government. Outbreak of severe acute respiratory syndrome (SARS) at Amoy Gardens, Kowloon Bay, Hong Kong. Main findings of the investigation. http://www.info.gov.hk/info/ap/pdf/amoy_e.pdf (accessed Aug 25, 2003).

25. WHO b. First data on stability and resistance of SARS coronavirus compiled by members of WHO laboratory network. Published online, 4 May 2003. http://www.who.int/csr/sars/survival.

26. Booth CM, Matukas LM, Tomlinson GA, *et al.* Clinical features and short-term outcomes of 144 patients with SARS in the Greater Toronto area. *JAMA* 2003;**289**:2801–2809.

27. Lipsitch M, Cohen T, Cooper B, *et al.* Transmission dynamics and control of severe acute respiratory syndrome. *Science* 2003;**300**:1966–1970.

28. Seto WH, Tsang D, Yung RW, *et al.* Effectiveness of precautions against droplets and contact in prevention of nosocomial transmission of severe acute respiratory syndrome (SARS). *Lancet* 2003;**361**:1519–1520.

3

Virology of SARS

Paul KS Chan

On 16 April 2003, the World Health Organization (WHO) announced that a novel coronavirus is the cause of the global outbreak of severe acute respiratory syndrome (SARS). The success and speed in identification of the culprit is a result of an unprecedented international collaboration involving 13 virus laboratories from 10 countries.[1,2] WHO and the network of laboratories have decided to dedicate their detection and characterization of the culprit virus to Dr. Carlo Urbani, who was the first WHO officer to detect the outbreak in Vietnam and later died of the infection.[3,4]

In 1882, Heinrich Koch, a German bacteriologist, set out four postulates for proving the etiological association between an infectious disease and its causative agent. This novel coronavirus fulfils these gold standard criteria. Firstly, the organism must be found in all cases. It has been shown that all SARS cases had serological evidence of infection with the novel coronavirus.[5-7] Secondly, it must be isolated from the host and grown in pure culture. The novel coronavirus has been isolated from post-mortem lung tissues of fatal SARS cases, and pure culture was grown from monkey kidney cells.[5-7] The third and fourth postulates require the reproduction of the original disease when the organism is introduced to a susceptible host, and it must be found in the experimental infected host. Cynomolgus macaques *(Macaca fascicularis)* inoculated with the novel coronavirus, isolated from a fatal SARS case, developed lung pathologies indistinguishable from those observed in fatal human SARS cases. The infected macaques showed seroconversion, and it was possible to isolate the viruses from nasal and throat secretions, and stool samples.[8,9] With these evidences, it is appropriate to refer to the novel coronavirus as SARS-associated coronavirus (SARS-CoV).

CORONAVIRUS

Coronavirus is a group of common pathogens that infects a variety of mammals and birds worldwide. Coronaviridae and Arteriviridae are the two families under the order Nidovirales. The family *Coronaviridae* comprises two genera, coronavirus and torovirus. The genus coronavirus has previously been divided into three groups, with little or no antigenic cross-reactivity. Mammalian coronaviruses form group I and group II, and avian coronaviruses form group III. Human coronaviruses (HCoVs)

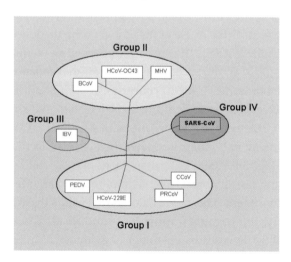

Fig. 1 Phylogenetic relationship of coronaviruses. Group I: canine coronavirus, CCoV; human coronavirus 229E, HCoV-229E; porcine epidemic diarrhea virus, PEDV; porcine respiratory coronavirus, PRCoV. Group II: bovine coronavirus, BCoV; human coronavirus OC43, HCoV-OC43; murine hepatitis virus, MHV. Group III, infectious bronchitis virus, IBV. Group IV: severe acute respiratory syndrome-associated coronavirus, SARS-CoV.

are found both in group I (HCoV-229E) and group II (HCoV-OC43). Results from phylogenetic analyses indicate that the newly identified SARS-CoV is distinct from the three groups of previously characterized coronaviruses. The amino acid homology between SARS-CoV and known coronaviruses ranges from 40% to 68% for non-structural proteins (protease, polymerase and helicase), and only 18% to 40% for structural proteins (spike, envelope, membrane and nucleocapsid).[10,11] The newly identified SARS-CoV should form the fourth group within the genus coronavirus. The genome of SARS-CoV appears to be between the cat and human species, and is more closely related to group II than to groups I or III coronaviruses (Fig. 1).

MORPHOLOGY

The virions of coronaviruses appear as round or elliptical particles with moderate pleomorphism. The virions range from 60 nm to 220 nm in diameter, with club-like projections evenly distributed over the circumference of the viral envelope. The name coronavirus originated from this "crown-like" surface halo formed by the spike (S) glycoproteins. SARS-CoV shares a similar morphology, except for a shorter anchor of the S glycoproteins, providing an easily recognizable feature to distinguish it from other coronaviruses (Fig. 2). In addition to S glycoproteins, membrane (M) glycoproteins and small envelope (E) proteins also constitute the viral envelope. Some groups II and III coronaviruses possess hemagglutinin-esterase (HE) glycoproteins that appear as short spikes on the virions. HE glycoproteins are not found in SARS-CoV. Inside the viral envelope is the internal core-shell composed of M glycoproteins and nucleocapsid (N) phosphoproteins. The RNA genome is associated with N phosphoproteins to form a long, flexible, helical nucleocapsid, enveloped by the internal core-shell (Fig. 3).

GENOME

The family *Coronaviridae* is characterized by a monopartite, single-stranded, plus-sense, capped, polyadenylated RNA genome ranging from 27 to 32 kilo-nucleotides in length.[12] All the coronaviruses share the same order of gene arrangement for the five major open reading frames (ORFs): polymerase-spike-envelope-membrane-nucleocapsid (5'-*Pol*-S-E-M-N-3'),

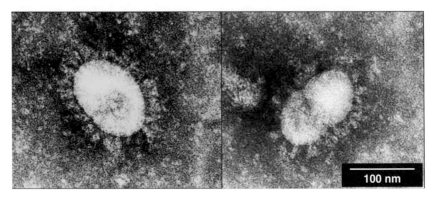

Fig. 2 Morphology of severe acute respiratory syndrome-associated coronavirus (SARS-CoV). The CUHK-W1 isolate was grown in African green monkey kidney cell monolayer. Cell culture supernatant was collected after four days of incubation when 90% of cells showed cytopathic effects. Cell culture supernatant was coated on a formvar-carbon grid and stained with 2% phosphotungstic acid for electron microscopy. Virions appear as pleomorphic ovoid and ellipsoid particles with club-like projections lining over the circumference giving rise to a "crown-like" appearance. The anchor of the surface spikes is shorter then other coronaviruses.

and with short untranslated regions (UTRs) at both termini. The reported full genomes of SARS-CoV range from 29–705 (Sin2677, GenBank accession number AY283795) to 29–757 (GZ01, GenBank accession number AY278489) nucleotides in length, and display the typical gene arrangement of coronaviruses, thus fulfilling one of the fundamental criteria for being a member of the family *Coronaviridae*. SARS-CoV does not contain the HE-encoding gene that is present between ORF 1b and S in some coronaviruses.

LIFE CYCLE

Coronaviruses bind to the plasma membrane of susceptible cells via S glycoproteins. For some coronaviruses, but not SARS-CoV, HE glycoproteins also function in virus entry. Coronaviruses can enter susceptible cells by acidic pH-dependent endocytosis or by pH-independent fusion at the plasma membrane.[13] It is not known which pathway predominates in SARS-CoV. Little is known about how the virus uncoats and releases its RNA genome into the cytoplasm, where the whole replication cycle takes

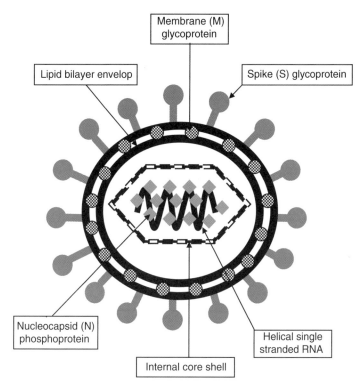

Fig. 3 Structure of coronaviruses.

place. Like other plus-sense RNA viruses, coronaviruses do not package with RNA-dependent RNA polymerase. Thus, RNA-dependent RNA polymerase has to be synthesized first, which then functions in transcripting the genomic as well as a nested set of subgenomic mRNAs. As observed in other coronaviruses, SARS-CoV utilizes genomic RNA for the translation of RNA-dependent RNA polymerase, whereas other structural and non-structural proteins are translated from subgenomic mRNAs.[10,11] As expected for coronaviruses in general, the nested set of subgenomic mRNA of SARS-CoV also shares a common 3′-coterminal, and each with a 5′-leader derived from the genomic 5′-leader sequence. The 5′-leader, also known as transcription regulating sequences (TRSs), of SARS-CoV is about 65–72 nucleotides in length and contains a conserved core sequence of 5′-AAACGAAC-3′. Within the SARS-CoV genome, the conserved core sequence of TRS appears six times in the genome in addition to the site at the 5′-termini. This predicts the presence of at least six major subgenomic mRNAs, of which five have been confirmed by Northern hybridization.[10] It is expected that more subgenomic mRNAs of smaller sizes or of less abundance exist. The first ORF from the 5' end (ORF 1 or *rep* gene) comprises approximately two-thirds of the SARS-CoV genome, and is predicted to encode for a precursor polyprotein with a protease domain (ORF 1a or *pro* gene) and a polymerase domain (ORF 1b or *pol* gene).[10,11] The S glycoprotein is co-translationally inserted into the rough endoplasmic reticulum and glycosylated with N-linked glycans. Some coronaviruses have their S glycoproteins cleaved into S1 and S2 subunits. This cleavage is probably not involved in SARS-CoV, as the basic amino acid cleavage site used by other coronaviruses does not exist

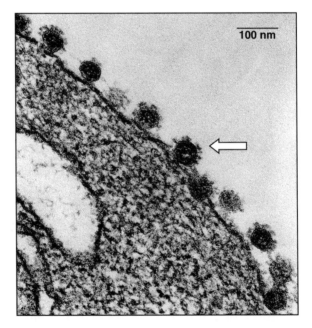

Fig. 4 Budding of severe acute respiratory syndrome-associated coronavirus (SARS-CoV). The CUHK-W1 isolate was grown in African green monkey kidney cell monolayer. Infected cells were collected after three days of incubation when 50% of cells showed cytopathic effects. Cell pellet was fixed with 2.5% of glutaldehyde and ultra-thin sections were prepared for electron microscopy. Arrow indicates a mature virion that has acquired its envelope and the associated glycoproteins through budding within the cisternae of the endoplasmic reticulum.

in the SARS-CoV genome.[10] Although the overall sequence conservation is low, the predicted E, M and N proteins of SARS-CoV contain conserved motifs found in other coronaviruses. The packaging of SARS-CoV is believed to be the same as for other coronaviruses. The N phosphoproteins bind to newly synthesized genomic RNA to form a helical nucleocapsid, which then interacts with M and E proteins within the endoplasmic reticulum and the Golgi complex. Virus budding is first detected in a specialized compartment located between the endoplasmic reticulum and the Golgi[14–16] (Fig. 4). Virions contained inside these smooth-walled vesicles are released by exocytosis (Fig. 5). Apparently, budding of virions does not occur on the plasma membrane.

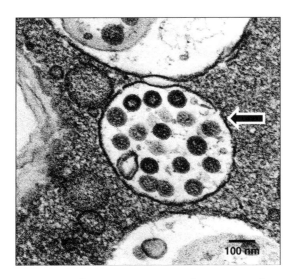

100 nm

Fig. 5 Mature virions of severe acute respiratory syndrome-associated coronavirus (SARS-CoV) inside an intracytoplasmic vesicle. The CUHK-W1 isolate was grown in African green monkey kidney cell monolayer. Infected cells were collected after three days of incubation when 50% of cells showed cytopathic effects. Cell pellet was fixed with 2.5% of glutaldehyde and ultra-thin sections were prepared for electron microscopy. Arrow indicates an intracytoplasmic vesicle containing a pouch of mature virions. This pouch of virions will be released from the infected cell by exocytosis accomplished by fusion between the smooth-walled vesicle and the plasma membrane.

SEQUENCE VARIABILITY

There are three possible mechanisms for coronaviruses to generate genetic heterogeneity. Firstly, like in other RNA viruses, random mutations take place as a result of high error frequency (about one per 10 000 nucleotides) of the RNA-dependent RNA polymerase.[17] The second mechanism involves the recombination of RNA genomes from different strains of the same species,[18,19] or from strains derived from different species.[20,21] The third mechanism involves the deletion of a stretch of nucleotides either as a result of recombination or other mechanisms.[22,23]

Up till now, the available sequence data of SARS-CoV have been derived from isolates obtained during the early phase of the global outbreak. So far, more than 20 full genome sequences of SARS-CoV have been published in GenBank. Comparison of the 14 full genome sequences obtained from northern and southern China, Hong Kong, Singapore, Vietnam and Toronto suggests the existence of two genotypes.[24] The first genotype represented by the Urbani (GenBank accession number AY278741) and TOR2 (GenBank accession number AY274119) isolates are epidemiologically linked to the hotel M in Hong Kong. The second genotype represented by the CUHK-W1 (GenBank accession number AY278554), GZ01 (GenBank accession number AY278489) and BJ01 (GenBank accession number AY278488) isolates are not related to the hotel M in Hong Kong. The two genotypes can be distinguished at four loci, suggesting that certain signature sequences of SARS-CoV can be used for contact tracing and delineating the source of infection (Fig. 6).

The stability of nucleotide sequences of the S glycoprotein gene has been examined in six isolates obtained from patients who acquired the infection from the same source.[25] The index case (patient X) of this cluster acquired the infection from the hotel M in Hong Kong, and was the source of the first major outbreak in Hong Kong.[26] The results show that despite the high error frequency expected for RNA polymerases, the sequences over the 3768-nucleotide long S glycoprotein encoding region were found to be identical for all the isolates. In the same study,[25] the full genome sequences of two representative isolates collected in the early phase of the outbreak in Hong Kong were compared. The first isolate designated as CUHK-Su10 (GenBank accession number AY282752) was obtained from the mother of the index case (patient X). The second isolate (CUHK-W1, GenBank accession number AY278554) was obtained from another

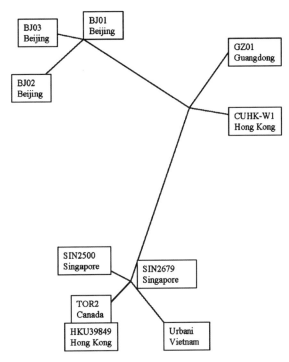

Fig. 6 Phylogenetic relationship of representative severe acute respiratory syndrome-associated coronavirus (SARS-CoV) isolates.

patient who acquired the infection directly from Shenzhen, China in early March. Altogether, 10 nucleotide differences between CUHK-Su10 and CUHK-W1 were observed, and these two isolates correspond respectively to each of the two genotypes as described by Ruan *et al.*[24] These sequence data indicates that there were at least two separate sources of infection present at the beginning of the SARS outbreak in Hong Kong. While sequence variability of isolates from different sources is extremely small with respect to expected error frequency of RNA-dependent RNA polymerases, signature sequences with epidemiological significance can be identified.

TROPISM

The S glycoprotein is the most critical determinant for tropism of coronaviruses. The S glycoprotein comprises three structural parts: a large external domain, a transmembrane domain and a carboxyl terminal cytoplasmic domain. The large external domain can be divided into two subdomains S1 and S2. S1 forms the globular portion of the spikes and is responsible for receptor binding. The S1 of murine hepatitis virus binds to the murine carcinoembryonic antigen-related cell adhesion molecules (mCEACAMs or CD66a), previously known as murine biliary glycoproteins (BGPs) that expressed in the liver, gastrointestinal tract, macrophages, and B cells.[27,28] The S1 of transmissible gastroenteritis virus (TGEV), a porcine coronavirus, binds to porcine aminopeptidase N that is expressed widely on many cell types, including respiratory and enteric epithelial cells, neuronal and glial cells.[29] The common human coronavirus HCoV-229E,[30] but not HCoV-OC43, utilizes the membrane-bound metalloproteinase, aminopeptidase N (CD13) as a receptor for cell entry. CD13 is highly expressed in human tissues, including lungs, immune cells, and activated vascular endothelium at the sites of inflammation.

It is difficult to predict the receptor or the tropism of SARS-CoV based on our knowledge of previously known coronaviruses, since the S glycoprotein of SARS-CoV only shows 20–27% amino acid sequence homology with other coronaviruses.[10] Therefore, one cannot infer CD13, the cellular receptor for HCoV-229E, as the receptor for SARS-CoV. Our studies on tropism for SARS-CoV do not support CD13 to be the receptor for SARS-CoV.

Our data from post-mortem materials indicate that SARS-CoV has a limited *in vivo* tissue tropism. Viruses have only been isolated from lungs and intestinal tissues. *In situ* hybridization using SARS-CoV specific probes revealed positive signals only from pneumocytes and enterocytes. Pneumocytes and enterocytes were also the only cell types where viral particles can be found under the electron microscope.

Since lymphopenia has been observed in a majority of patients,[31] it is important to verify whether SARS-CoV is lymphotropic. We have examined peripheral blood mononuclear cells collected from patients within 10 days following the onset of illness. Our results from reverse-transcription polymerase chain reaction and *in situ* hybridization do not show evidence of *de novo* infection in peripheral blood mononuclear cells. In connection with this, we have examined several CD13-positive hemic cell lines and none of them can support the replication of SARS-CoV. So far, evidence for SARS-CoV being lymphotropic is lacking.

The possibility of SARS-CoV being neurotropic has been raised since RNA sequences of HCoV-299E and HCoV-OC43 have been found in human brain tissues and cerebrospinal fluid.[32–34] We have detected SARS-CoV RNA from the cerebrospinal fluid of a patient who developed neurological illness during the course of SARS-CoV infection. The possibility of SARS-CoV being neurotropic cannot be ignored.

Unlike HCoV-299E and HCoV-OC43 that are difficult to isolate *in vitro*, SARS-CoV is readily isolated from African green monkey kidney (Vero) cells or their subclones, including Vero E6, Vero 118 and Vero 76. Most positive clinical specimens show characteristic diffuse refractile rounding cytopathic effects after 2–4 days of incubation (Fig. 7).

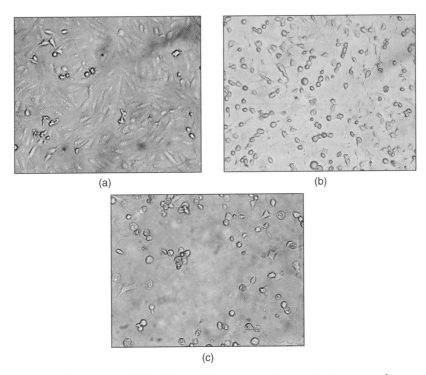

(a)   (b)

(c)

Fig. 7 *In vitro* cytopathic effects of severe acute respiratory syndrome-associated coronavirus (SARS-CoV). African green monkey kidney cell monolayer inoculated with the CUHK-W1 isolate. (a) Cell monolayer before inoculation of viruses. (b) After three days of incubation, about 50% of cells show refractile rounding cytopathic effects that are characteristic of SARS-CoV infection in African green monkey cell monolayer. (c) After four days of incubation, most cells have detached from the monolayer. The remaining cells show cytopathic effects and will be detached within 6–12 hours.

ANTIVIRAL SUSCEPTIBILITY

Until recently, coronaviruses remain a cause of self-limiting common cold and have never been a focus for antiviral development. At the onset of the epidemics in March 2003, ribavirin has been used for SARS cases based on its broad spectrum of antiviral activity.[35] Ribavirin is a purine nucleoside analogue, which inhibits the enzyme inosine monophosphate dehydrogenase. Ribavirin has an *in vitro* inhibitory effect on the replication of respiratory syncytial virus, influenza and parainfluenza. In most countries, ribavirin is licensed for the treatment of respiratory syncytial virus, and hepatitis C infection in combination with interferon. High dose ribavirin is also recommended for viral hemorrhagic fever. Subsequently, the *in vitro* effect of ribavirin on SARS-CoV has been examined by Huggins *et al.* at the United States Army Medical Research Institute of Infectious Diseases. It was found that ribavirin has no inhibitory effect on SARS-CoV both by cell protection assay at a low multiplicity of infection and by plaque reduction assay based on Vero 76 and Vero E6 cell systems.

Glycyrrhizin, an active component derived from liquorice roots, has been shown to produce antiviral effect against SARS-CoV *in vitro*.[36] Glycyrrhizin has been used to treat human immunodeficiency virus type 1 and hepatitis C virus infections. Using the Vero cell system, glycyrrhizin showed a selective index of 67, which is defined as the ratio of concentration of a compound that reduces cell viability to 50% to the concentration of that compound needed to inhibit the cytopathic effect to 50% of the control values. The antiviral effect of glycyrrhizin was most effective when the drug was present both during and after the adsorption period, suggesting inhibition at viral entry as well as replication. The study also examined other drugs and found no antiviral effect for ribavirin and mycophenolic acid; and a low selective index (6 and 12) for inhibitors of orotidine monophosphate decarboxylase, 6-azauridine and pyrazofurin. The mechanism for antiviral activity of glycyrrhizin is not known. Glycyrrhizin has multiple interactions with cellular pathways, including the protein kinase C, casein kinase II, transcription activator protein I and nuclear factor κB. Glycyrrhizin also upregulates inducible nitrous oxide synthase, resulting in the production of nitrous oxide in macrophages.[37] It has been shown that nitrous oxide has inhibitory effects on RNA virus replication.[38]

The *in vitro* antiviral effects of interferons have been examined by Cinatl *et al.*[39] Based on the Vero cell culture system, interferon β was found to produce antiviral effects on SARS-CoV when applied prophylat-ically or after infection. However, the use of interferon, an immunomodu-lating agent, for treating SARS patients requires further considerations as the current observation suggests that the pathogenesis of SARS may have a strong immune-mediated component.

ORIGIN

Most coronaviruses can only establish infection in one host species. Although the two prototype human coronaviruses (HCoV-229E and HCoV-OC43) account for about 30% of common colds, they rarely cause lower respiratory tract infection.[40–42] The benign nature of human coron-aviruses is in contrast to infections seen in livestock and poultry that often result in devastating respiratory or enteric diseases.[43–47] This raises the suspicion that the outbreak of SARS in humans was started off by a cross-species infection. It is clear from genome sequence data that SARS-CoV is neither a mutant nor a recombinant of coronaviruses known to exist in humans or animal species. There are also no footprints suggestive of arti-ficial genetic manipulations. The SARS-CoV, or its immediate ancestor, has probably established a long history of unrecognized infection in one or more animal species. The recent outbreak in humans was probably a result of a cross-species infection with a prior sequence mutation, deletion or recombination leading to a dramatic change in its species specificity.

A research team in southern China announced that they have found SARS-CoV from masked palm civets (*Paguma larvata*), raccoon dogs (*Nyctereutes procyonoides*) and probably from about half-a-dozen species of animals in a market at Dongmen in Shenzhen, located in the southern Chinese province of Guangdong, where the SARS outbreak first emerged in November 2002.[48–50] Compared with the coronavirus sequences found in civet cats, the SARS-CoV found in humans has a 29-nucleotide deletion in an ORF with unknown function. However, a research team at the China Agriculture University in Beijing did not find any trace of SARS-CoV from their survey on 732 animals from 54 wild and 11 domestic species, including palm civets from southern China. Instead, the team iso-lated a different coronavirus from civets with about 77% sequence homol-ogy to SARS-CoV.

The hypothesis that the SARS-CoV infecting humans originated from edible animal species(s) is supported by the finding of a high proportion

(9/23) of early SARS cases being food handlers, and people living close to markets are also over-represented.[49]

While the origin of the novel SARS-CoV is still a mystery, the virus has suddenly disappeared after a global epidemic of 4 months. Although every corner of the world has made all possible efforts to interrupt the transmission of SARS-CoV in humans, the reason for its disappearance, at least temporarily, may involve factors other than human efforts. To understand how an emerging infection can be extinguished is as important as tracing its origin. There is still a tremendous body of knowledge to be revealed from the evolution of SARS-CoV, the first fatal emerging infection in this century.

OTHER VIRUSES

While there is little doubt about the etiological association between the novel coronavirus and SARS, it is worth noting that another recently identified virus, the human metapneumovirus (hMPV), has also been found in patients with clinical presentations similar to those described for SARS. Among the first cluster of SARS cases in Canada, hMPV was detected from five of six patients.[51] In that series, coronavirus was also detected from five of six patients, and four were coinfected with hMPV and coronavirus. A high prevalence of hMPV was also observed among the first cluster of SARS patients seen in the Prince of Wales Hospital, where the first SARS outbreak in Hong Kong occurred. Of the 48 SARS patients investigated, 52% had hMPV isolated from nasopharyngeal aspirate samples.[52] Just a few days before the outbreak of SARS was noticed, a previously healthy adult was admitted to the Prince of Wales Hospital. The patient developed acute pneumonia while staying in southern China. He did not respond to antibiotics and died suddenly eight days after the onset of illness. Human metapneumovirus was isolated from postmortem lung tissue, whereas no coronavirus or other pathogens could be found.[53] Foulongne et al.[54] from France also reported the detection of hMPV from a patient with clinical suspicion of SARS [GenBank accession number: AY291314]. An outbreak of acute illness in a long term care facility in South Western British Columbia occurred from July till August 2003. Although the outbreak was clinically not compatible with the previously described SARS, the possibility of re-emergence of SARS was a real concern at that time. Of interest, the preliminary investigations showed four individuals were positive for hMPV and two of them were also infected with coronavirus.

Human metapneumovirus (hMPV) was first identified in 2001 from children with respiratory tract diseases.[55] It is now known that hMPV infection is prevalent worldwide and associated with a wild spectrum of respiratory illnesses.[56–61] It is likely that a proportion of hMPV infections can mimic SARS-CoV infections, and may account for some cases that have a clinical diagnosis of SARS. Coinfection of hMPV with respiratory syncytial virus (RSV) in infants has been suggested to be a factor influencing the severity of bronchiolitis.[61] Whether coinfection with hMPV and SARS-CoV would result in more adverse outcome deserves further investigations. The diagnosis for hMPV infection is far more difficult than for SARS-CoV. The virus is difficult to grow and serological test is not widely available. It is expected that more time and efforts will be needed before a clearer role of hMPV in SARS can be elucidated.

REFERENCES

1. WHO. A multicentre collaboration to investigate the cause of severe acute respiratory syndrome. *Lancet* 2003;**361**:1730–33.

2. WHO. SARS virus identified. *Bull World Health Organ* 2003A;**81**:384.

3. Reilley B, Van Herp M, Sermand D. SARS and Carlo Urbani. *N Engl J Med* 2003;**348**:1951–52.

4. WHO. WHO frontline worker dies of severe acute respiratory syndrome (SARS). *Bull World Health Organ* 2003B;**81**:384.

5. Ksiazek TG, Erdman D, Goldsmith CS, *et al.* A novel coronavirus associated with severe acute respiratory syndrome. *N Engl J Med* **348**:1953–66.

6. Peiris JS, Lai ST, Poon LL. Coronavirus as a possible cause of severe acute respiratory syndrome. *Lancet* 2003;**361**:1319–25.

7. Drosten C, Gunther S, Preiser W, *et al.* Identification of a novel coronavirus in patients with severe acute respiratory syndrome. *N Engl J Med* 2003;**348**:1967–76.

8. Fouchier RA, Kuiken T, Schutten M, *et al.* Aetiology: Koch's postulates fulfilled for SARS virus. *Nature* 2003;**423**:240.

9. Kuiken T, Fouchier RA, Schutten M, *et al.* Newly discovered coronavirus as the primary cause of severe acute respiratory syndrome. *Lancet* 2003;**362**:263–70.

10. Rota PA, Oberste MS, Monroe SS, *et al.* Characterization of a novel coronavirus associated with severe acute respiratory syndrome. *Science* 2003;**300**:1394–98.

11. Marra MA, Jones SJ, Astell CR, *et al.* The genome sequence of the SARS-associated coronavirus. *Science* 2003;**300**:1399–04.

12. Lai MM, Cavanagh D. The molecular biology of coronaviruses. *Adv Virus Res* 1997;**48**:1–100.

13. Kooi C, Cervin M, Anderson R. Differentiation of acid-pH-dependent and -nondependent entry pathways for mouse hepatitis virus. *Virology* 1991;**180**:108–19.

14. Klumperman J, Locker JK, Meijer A, *et al.* Coronavirus M proteins accumulate in the Golgi complex beyond the site of virion budding. *J Virol* 1994;**68**:6523–34.

15. Tooze J, Tooze S, Warren G. Replication of coronavirus MHV-A59 in sac- cells: Determination of the first site of budding of progeny virions. *Eur J Cell Biol* 1984;**33**:281–93.

16. Tooze J, Tooze SA. Infection of AtT20 murine pituitary tumour cells by mouse hepatitis virus strain A59: Virus budding is restricted to the Golgi region. *Eur J Cell Biol* 1985;**37**:203–12.

17. Steinhauer DA, Holland JJ. Direct method for quantitation of extreme polymerase error frequencies at selected single base sites in viral RNA. *J Virol* 1986;**57**:219–28.

18. Makino S, Keck JG, Stohlman SA, Lai MM. High-frequency RNA recombination of murine coronaviruses. *J Virol* 1986;**57**:729–37.

19. Makino S, Fleming JO, Keck JG. RNA recombination of coronaviruses: Localization of neutralizing epitopes and neuropathogenic determinants on the carboxyl terminus of peplomers. *Proc Natl Acad Sci USA* 1987;**84**:6567–71.

20. Herrewegh AA, Smeenk I, Horzinek MC, *et al.* Feline coronavirus type II strains 79-1683 and 79-1146 originate from a double recombination between feline coronavirus type I and canine coronavirus. *J Virol* 1998;**72**:4508–14.

21. Wesley RD. The S gene of canine coronavirus, strain UCD-1, is more closely related to the S gene of transmissible gastroenteritis virus than to that of feline infectious peritonitis virus. *Virus Res* 1999;**61**:145–52.

22. Rowe CL, Fleming JO, Nathan MJ, *et al.* Generation of coronavirus spike deletion variants by high-frequency recombination at regions of predicted RNA secondary structure. *J Virol* 1997;**71**:6183–90.

23. Rowe CL, Baker SC, Nathan MJ, Fleming JO. Evolution of mouse hepatitis virus: Detection and characterization of spike deletion variants during persistent infection. *J Virol* 1997A;**71**:2959–69.

24. Ruan YJ, Wei CL, Ee AL, *et al.* Comparative full-length genome sequence analysis of 14 SARS coronavirus isolates and common mutations associated with putative origins of infection. *Lancet* 2003;**361**:1779–85.

25. Tsui SK, Chim SS, Lo YM. Coronavirus genomic-sequence variations and the epidemiology of the severe acute respiratory syndrome. *N Engl J Med* 2003;**349**:187–88.

26. Lee N, Hui D, Wu A, *et al.* A major outbreak of severe acute respiratory syndrome in Hong Kong. *N Engl J Med* 2003;**348**:1986–94.

27. Williams RK, Jiang GS, Holmes KV. Receptor for mouse hepatitis virus is a member of the carcinoembryonic antigen family of glycoproteins. *Proc Natl Acad Sci USA* 1991;**88**: 5533–36.

28. Tsai JC, Zelus BD, Holmes KV, Weiss SR. The N-terminal domain of the murine coronavirus spike glycoprotein determines the CEACAM1 receptor specificity of the virus strain. *J Virol* 2003;**77**:841–50.

29. Kusters JG, Niesters HG, Lenstra JA, *et al.* Phylogeny of antigenic variants of avian coronavirus IBV. *Virology* 1989;**169**:217–21.

30. Bonavia A, Zelus BD, Wentworth DE, Talbot PJ, Holmes KV. Identification of a receptor-binding domain of the spike glycoprotein of human coronavirus HCoV-229E. *J Virol* 2003;**77**:2530–38.

31. Wong RS, Wu A, To KF, *et al.* Haematological manifestations in patients with severe acute respiratory syndrome: Retrospective analysis. *BMJ* 2003;**326**:1358–62.

32. Cristallo A, Gambaro F, Biamonti G, *et al.* Human coronavirus polyadenylated RNA sequences in cerebrospinal fluid from multiple sclerosis patients. *New Microbiol* 1997;**20**:105–14.

33. Dessau RB, Lisby G, Frederiksen JL. Coronaviruses in spinal fluid of patients with acute monosymptomatic optic neuritis. *Acta Neurol Scand* 1999;**100**:88–91.

34. Stewart JN, Mounir S, Talbot PJ. Human coronavirus gene expression in the brains of multiple sclerosis patients. *Virology* 1992;**191**:502–5.

35. Koren G, King S, Knowles S, Phillips E. Ribavirin in the treatment of SARS: A new trick for an old drug? *CMAJ* 2003;**168**:1289–92.

36. Cinatl J, Morgenstern B, Bauer G, *et al.* Glycyrrhizin, an active component of liquorice roots, and replication of SARS-associated coronavirus. *Lancet* 2003;**361**:2045–6.

37. Jeong HG, Kim JY. Induction of inducible nitric oxide synthase expression by 18beta-glycyrrhetinic acid in macrophages. *FEBS Lett* 2002;**513**:208–12.

38. Lin YL, Huang YL, Ma SH. Inhibition of Japanese encephalitis virus infection by nitric oxide: Antiviral effect of nitric oxide on RNA virus replication. *J Virol* 1997;**71**:5227–35.

39. Cinatl J, Morgenstern B, Bauer G, *et al.* Treatment of SARS with human interferons. *Lancet* 2003A;**362**:293–4.

40. Bradburne AF, Bynoe ML, Tyrrell DA. Effects of a "new" human respiratory virus in volunteers. *Br Med J* 1967;**3**:767–9.

41. Isaacs D, Flowers D, Clarke JR, *et al.* Epidemiology of coronavirus respiratory infections. *Arch Dis Child* 1983;**58**:500–3.

42. Monto AS. Medical reviews. Coronaviruses. *Yale J Biol Med* 1974;**47**:234–51.

43. Woods RD, Wesley RD. Transmissible gastroenteritis coronavirus carrier sow. *Adv Exp Med Biol* 1998;**440**:641–7.

44. Laude H, Van Reeth K, Pensaert M. Porcine respiratory coronavirus: Molecular features and virus-host interactions. *Vet Res* 1993;**24**:125–50.

45. Adams NR, Ball RA, Hofstad MS. Intestinal lesions in transmissible enteritis of turkeys. *Avian Dis* 1970;**14**:392–9.

46. Zanella A, Lavazza A, Marchi R, *et al.* Avian infectious bronchitis: Characterization of new isolates from Italy. *Avian Dis* 2003;**47**:180–5.

47. Halbur PG, Pallares FJ, Opriessnig T, *et al.* Pathogenicity of three isolates of porcine respiratory coronavirus in the USA. *Vet Rec* 2003;**152**:358–61.

48. Cyranoski D, Abbott A. Virus detectives seek source of SARS in China's wild animals. *Nature* 2003;**423**:467.

49. Normile D, Enserink M. SARS in China. Tracking the roots of a killer. *Science* 2003;**301**:297–9.

50. Pearson H, Clarke T, Abbott A, *et al*. SARS: What have we learned? *Nature* 2003;**424**:121–6.

51. Poutanea SM, Low DE, Henry B. Identification of severe acute respiratory syndrome in Canada. *N Engl J Med* 2003;**348**(20):1995–2005.

52. Chan PKS, Tam JS, Lam CW, *et al*. Detection of human metapneumovirus from patients with severe acute respiratory syndrome. *Emerg Infect Dis* 2003;**9**:1058–63.

53. Chan PKS, To KF, Wu A, *et al*. Human metapneumovirus-associated a typical pneumonia and SARS. *Emerg Infect Dis* 2004;**10**:497–500.

54. van den Hoogen BG, de Jong JC, Groen J, *et al*. A newly discovered human pneumovirus isolated from young children with respiratory tract disease. *Nat Med* 2001;**7**:719–24.

55. Jartti T, van den Hoogen B, Garofalo RP, *et al*. Metapneumovirus and acute wheezing in children. *Lancet* 2002;**360**:1393–4.

56. Freymouth F, Vabret A, Legrand L, *et al*. Presence of the new human metapneumovirus in French children with bronchiolitis. *Pediatr Infect Dis J* 2003;**22**:92–4.

57. Stockton J, Stephenson I, Fleming D, Zambon M. Human metapneumovirus as a cause of community-acquired respiratory illness. *Emerg Infect Dis* 2002;**8**:897–901.

58. Boivin G, De Serres G, Cote S, *et al*. Virological features and clinical manifestations associated with human metapneumovirus: A new paramyxovirus responsible for acute respiratory-tract infections in all age groups. *J Infect Dis* 2002;**186**:1330–4.

59. Osterhaus A, Fouchier R. Human metapneumovirus in the community. *Lancet* 2003;**361**:890–1.

60. Falsey AR, Erdman D, Anderson LJ, Walsh EE. Human metapneumovirus infections in young and elderly adults. *J Infect Dis* 2003;**187**:785–90.

61. Greensill J, McNamara PS, Dove W, *et al*. Human metapneumovirus in severe respiratory syncytial virus bronchiolitis. *Emerg Infect Dis* 2003;**9**:372–5.

4

Clinical Presentations and Manifestations of SARS

Nelson Lee, WK Leung

INTRODUCTION

Severe Acute Respiratory Syndrome (SARS) is a newly emerging infectious disease caused by a novel *coronavirus*.[1] From February to June 2003, there were over 8400 cases reported worldwide, with more than 900 deaths and significant morbidity in many patients.[2] In the most severe cases, respiratory failure and acute respiratory distress syndrome (ARDS) ensued that might require the use of mechanical ventilation. Since the pathogen is highly contagious, persons suffering from SARS need to be promptly recognized and isolated. In this chapter, clinical presentations and manifestations, the typical clinical course and atypical presentations of SARS are highlighted and reviewed.

According to the case definition of SARS by the Centers for Disease Control (CDC), a "probable" case of SARS should meet the clinical criteria for *severe* respiratory illness of unknown etiology and epidemiologic criteria for exposure, with laboratory criteria either confirmed or undetermined (Table 1).[3] The presence of fever (>38°C), respiratory symptoms (e.g. cough, shortness of breath), and pneumonic changes on radiographs

Table 1 CDC Case Definitions of SARS[3]

Clinical Criteria
- Asymptomatic or mild respiratory illness
- Moderate respiratory illness
  - Temperature of >100.4°F (>38°C), and
  - One or more clinical findings of respiratory illness (e.g. cough, shortness of breath, difficulty in breathing, or hypoxia).
- Severe respiratory illness
  - Temperature of >100.4°F (>38°C), and
  - One or more clinical findings of respiratory illness (e.g. cough, shortness of breath, difficulty in breathing, or hypoxia), and
    - radiographic evidence of pneumonia, or
    - respiratory distress syndrome, or
    - autopsy findings consistent with pneumonia or respiratory distress syndrome without an identifiable cause.

Epidemiologic Criteria
- Travel (including transit in an airport) within 10 days of onset of symptoms to an area with current or previously documented or suspected community transmission of SARS (see Table below),
  or
- Close contact within 10 days of onset of symptoms with a person known or suspected to have SARS.

Laboratory Criteria
- Confirmed
  - Detection of antibody to SARS-associated coronavirus (SARS-CoV) in a serum sample, or
  - Detection of SARS-CoV RNA by RT-PCR confirmed by a second PCR assay, by using a second aliquot of the specimen and a different set of PCR primers, or
  - Isolation of SARS-CoV.
- Negative
  - Absence of antibody to SARS-CoV in a convalescent-phase serum sample obtained >28 days after symptom onset.
- Undetermined
  - Laboratory testing either not performed or incomplete.

Case Classification
- Probable case: meets the clinical criteria for severe respiratory illness of unknown etiology and epidemiologic criteria for exposure; laboratory criteria confirmed or undetermined.
- Suspect case: meets the clinical criteria for moderate respiratory illness of unknown etiology, and epidemiologic criteria for exposure; laboratory criteria confirmed or undetermined.

Continued

Table 1 *Continued*

Exclusion Criteria

A case may be excluded as a suspect or probable SARS case, if:

- An alternative diagnosis can fully explain the illness.
- The case has a convalescent-phase serum sampe (i.e. obtained >28 days after symptoms onset) which is negative for antibody to SARS-CoV.
- The case was reported on the basis of contact with an index case that was subsequently excluded as a case of SARS, provided other possible epidemiologic exposure criteria are not present.

---

or ARDS are classified as severe respiratory illness. "Suspect" cases are those who meet the clinical criteria for *moderate* respiratory illness of unknown etiology and epidemiologic criteria for exposure, with laboratory criteria either confirmed or undetermined. The presence of fever (>38°C) and respiratory symptoms, without pneumonic changes on chest radiographs are classified as a moderate respiratory illness. Cases are excluded only if an alternative explanation for the illness is found, or a convalescent-phase serology test for the SARS-associated coronavirus (SARS-CoV) being negative.[3] The WHO case definition for surveillance of SARS is similar.[2] While these case definitions remain important for epidemiological surveillance, isolation and management purposes, it was established based on retrospective clinical data of early SARS cases, irrespective of virological confirmation of *coronavirus* infection. Through the accumulation of clinical experiences and improvement in laboratory diagnosis of SARS-CoV, the characteristic clinical course of illness and atypical manifestations of SARS are now better recognized and described.

SYSTEMIC SYMPTOMS AND CLINICAL COURSE OF ILLNESS

The mean incubation period of SARS is estimated to be 6.4 days (95% confidence interval, 5.2–7.7 days), and the mean time from onset of clinical symptoms to hospital admission varied between 3 and 5 days.[9] The typical presentations of SARS described in different case series are summarized in Table 2[4-8]. In fact, non-specific systemic symptoms are usually the first manifestations of SARS. The majority of patients develop fever, myalgia, chills/rigor, non-productive cough, headache and dizziness

Table 2 Clinical Presentations of SARS in Different Case Series[4–8]

Clinical Features (%)	Hong Kong Lee N, et al.[4] (n = 138)	Toronto Booth CM, et al.[5] (n = 144)	Hong Kong Peiris JSM, et al.[6] (n = 50)	Guangzhou Wu W, et al.[7] (n = 96)	Singapore Hsu LY, et al.[8] (n = 20)
Fever	100	99.3	100	100	100
Chills/rigor	73.2	27.8	74	55.2	15
Myalgia	60.9	49.3	54	21.9	45
Cough	57.3	69.4	62	85.4	75
Dyspnoea	—	41.7	20	—	40
Headache	55.8	35.4	20	39.6	20
Dizziness	42.8	4.2	12	—	—
Sputum	29.0	4.9	—	66.7	—
Diarrhoea	19.6	23.6	10	—	25
Nausea & vomiting	19.6	19.4	20	—	35
Sore throat	23.2	12.5	20	—	25
Malaise	—	31.2	50	35.4	45

initially. Although fever >38°C was included in the case definition of SARS (which was a retrospective observation), a patient's temperature upon presentation may be <38°C or even normal. According to Booth's series from Toronto,[5] only 85% of their cases had fever >38°C documented on admission; the remaining 15% either reported fever prior to presentation or developed a temperature upon hospitalization. By day 4 of admission, only 28% of the cases remained febrile. Overall, 99.3% of patients reported that they had fever at some point of their illnesses. A similar observation was made by the Hong Kong investigators. Upon presentation to a SARS screening clinic, only 81% of cases developed a high fever, though all confirmed cases eventually fulfilled the case definition of SARS.[10] It was also noted by another group that a patient's fever initially improved after admission, but subsequently recurred at a mean of 8.9 (±3.1 SD) days.[6] Thus, a patients' fever pattern must be carefully monitored; absence of fever on presentation does not exclude the diagnosis of SARS.

The symptoms of chills, rigor and myalgia are prevalent on presentation. It is believed that these symptoms may represent viremia as in many other systemic viral illnesses (e.g. influenza). According to clinical observations, these symptoms gradually subside towards the end of the first week of illness, which corresponds to the decline in viral replication. In one study, the viral load of SARS-CoV was noted to increase progressively in respiratory secretions, stool and urine during the first week, and then declined after day 10 of illness.[6] Myalgia is associated with elevated serum creatinine phosphokinase (CPK) level in some cases,[4] but whether this represents a low grade myositis remains unclear. Other non-specific symptoms, such as dizziness, headache and malaise also appear to be very common complaints among patients suffering from SARS. In some cases, dizziness can be quite severe.[11] However, there is at present no convincing evidence to suggest SARS-CoV invaded the human central nervous system leading to these symptoms. Skin rash, lymphadenopathy and organomegaly are typically absent.[4]

Generally, the clinical course of SARS follows a triphasic pattern.[11,12] In Phase I or the viral replication phase (from symptoms onset to day 7–10 of illness), systemic symptoms are most prominent. At this stage, chest radiographs and/or CT scan of the thorax show mostly focal and slowly progressive pneumonic changes.[11-13] When the symptoms of viremia subside, there may even be a transient period of clinical improvement before the infection progresses to the second phase. In Phase II or the period of immunopathological damage, fever returns and the patient may experience shortness of breath. Many patients also develop watery diarrhea at this stage.[6] It has been estimated that 80% of patients progress to the second phase, at a mean of 7.4 days.[6] Chest radiographs show rapidly progressive multi-focal or bilateral air-space consolidation. The patient's conditions may change within 12 hours. Oxygen desaturation develops as the disease becomes more extensive. Interestingly, this phase is associated with a declining viral load.[6] Nonetheless, the majority of patients respond to supportive, as well as corticosteroid (+/− ribavirin) therapy[14,15]. Around 20–25% of cases would progress to Phase III, when severe respiratory failure and ARDS would ensue.[9,16,17] To conclude, it becomes clear that the presence of fever and occurrence of SARS-associated symptoms varies depending on the time of presentation. Careful follow-up of the entire disease course is mandatory.[10] Recognizing the characteristic triphasic pattern is also helpful when making a diagnosis of SARS.

RESPIRATORY MANIFESTATIONS

Respiratory illness is the major manifestation and complication of SARS. Dry cough is the presenting symptom of SARS in 57–85% of cases and sputum production is uncommon (Table 2). Interestingly, although human non-SARS associated coronaviruses usually produce the "common cold", coryza is a rare manifestation of SARS, suggesting major virologic and pathogenic differences between the two viruses. Though shortness of breath appears to be a distinguishing feature of SARS,[3,10] it usually occurs after the first week of illness, reflecting a more extensive pulmonary involvement and progressing to subsequent development of ARDS. Oxygen desaturation occurs at a mean of 9.1 days as the disease progresses.[6] Auscultation of the chest may reveal inspiratory crackles in the lung bases but wheezing is absent.[4] Since about 20% of patients had no evidence of air-space consolidation at the time of fever onset,[12] an initial normal chest radiograph does not exclude the diagnosis of SARS and follow-up imaging is usually necessary.[10] Radiologically, airspace consolidation is usually unilateral, focal and sometimes peripherally located in the first phase of viral replication.[12,13] In the second phase, pulmonary infiltrates become multifocal, bilateral and be even shifting. The shifting nature of radiographic shadows, and the timing of the second phase being coincident with seroconversion and reduction in viral load, suggest a immunologically mediated lung damage instead of direct cytolysis. In many cases, there are features resembling bronchiolitis obliterans organizing pneumonia (BOOP), an immune mediated disease which is responsive to corticosteroid therapy, as shown on CT scan of the thorax.[4,18]

Around 20–25% of patients eventually were found to develop severe respiratory failure and ARDS that necessitated ICU care, with or without mechanical ventilation.[4,6,16,17] In a pathology study of six serologically confirmed SARS cases, diffuse alveolar damage was the most common postmortem finding.[19] Morphological changes included bronchial epithelial denudation, loss of cilia, squamous metaplasia, giant-cell infiltrate, and increase in macrophages in the alveoli and interstitium of the lung. Alveolar pneumocytes showed cytomegaly with granular amphophilic cytoplasm. Electron microscopy revealed SARS-CoV viral particles in the cytoplasm of epithelial cells. Interestingly, hemophagocytosis was also observed, which supported the theory that cytokine dysregulation may partly account for the illness. On the other hand, it was found that higher intra-pulmonary viral loads were significantly associated with shorter periods of survival in another study, suggesting SARS-CoV might directly contribute to disease progression and death.[20]

It is recognized that 19–23% of cases required ICU admission.[16,17] The majority of the patients fulfilled the criteria for acute lung injury (ALI) or ARDS. ARDS was characterized by ease of derecruitment of alveoli and paucity of airway secretion, bronchospasm, or dynamic hyperinflation. In the Singapore series, mortality at 28 days was 10.1% for the entire cohort and 37% for ICU patients. The mortality of ICU patients at 13 weeks was 52.2%, which usually occurred late (≥7 days after ICU admission), and was attributed to complications related to severe ARDS, multiorgan failure, thromboembolic complications, or septicemic shock. In the Toronto series, the median interval between initial symptoms and admission to the ICU was 8 days (inter-quartile range IQR 5–10) days. Seventy-six percent of ICU cases required mechanical ventilation. The 28-day mortality for ICU cases was 34%, and for those requiring mechanical ventilation, 45%. Sixteen percent of patients still required mechanical ventilation at 28 days. Patients with lower acute physiology and chronic health evaluation (APCHE) II scores and higher baseline ratios of PaO_2 to fraction of inspired oxygen, were associated with earlier recovery. Advanced age (therefore usually involving the non-healthcare workers), preexisting diabetes mellitus, bilateral radiographic infiltrates on presentation, admission tachycardia, high neutrophil counts, elevated serum creatinine kinase (CPK) and lactate dehydrogenase (LDH) levels, were associated with more severe illness, poorer clinical outcome and death.[4,16,17,21] The high LDH possibly reflects more severe tissue damage, similar to the case of *Pneumocystis carinii* pneumonia, in which a higher LDH level was associated with a more severe disease.

Interestingly, pneumonthorax and pneumomediastinum, either spontaneous or associated with mechanical ventilation, were commonly encountered in critically ill SARS cases. In one report, 12% of seriously ill SARS patients developed spontaneous pneumomediastinum.[6] In different series, 20% of ICU patients and 34% of those being mechanically ventilated developed pneumothorax/pneumomediastinum.[16,17] The incidence of barotraumas was unusually high despite low-volume low-pressure mechanical ventilation.[12] The reason for this observation is unclear as chest radiographs did not demonstrate excessive hyperinflation or bullous lung disease. Based on histological examination, there is pulmonary edema with hyaline membrane formation and cellular fibromyxoid-organizing exudates in airspaces, suggesting that reduction in lung compliance may be partially responsible for the high incidence of barotrauma.

ENTERIC MANIFESTATIONS

Apart from respiratory symptoms, diarrhea is a common and important manifestation of SARS. In a retrospective analysis of the gastrointestinal symptoms and other clinical parameters of the first 138 confirmed SARS patients admitted for a major outbreak in Hong Kong, 28 (20.3%) presented with watery diarrhea,[4] and up to 38.4% patients had diarrhea symptoms during the course of the illness (Fig. 1).[22] In some patients, diarrhea and fever could be the only initial manifestation of SARS, even in the absence of pneumonia on radiograph.[23] Diarrhea was more frequently observed during the first 10 days of illness. The mean number of days with diarrhea was 3.7 ± 2.7, most of the diarrhea cases being self-limiting. In another report from Hong Kong, which included over 1400 patients,[9] up to 27% of the patients had diarrhea. In another Hong Kong series, watery diarrhea was present in up to 73% of cases after the first week of illness (mean 7.5 ± 2.3 days).[6]

Intestinal biopsies obtained by colonoscopy or during autopsy showed minimal inflammation or architectural disruption. However, ultrastructural studies showed the presence of viral particles (60–90 nm in size) within both small and large intestinal cells. Viral particles were

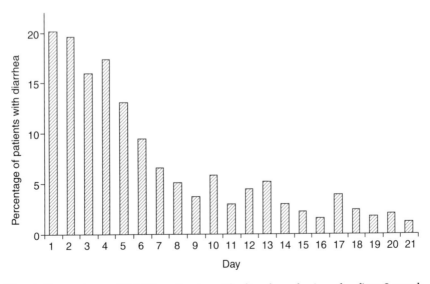

Fig. 1 Percentage of SARS patients with diarrhea during the first 3 week of illness.

confined to the epithelial cells, primarily in the apical surface enterocytes and rarely in the glandular epithelial cells. Intracellularly, viral particles were contained within dilated cytoplasmic vesicles consistent with a dilated endoplasmic reticulum. The vesicles containing the viral particles were often seen towards the apical cytoplasm. Clusters of coronavirus were also detected on the surface micro-villi, which may suggest virus leaving the luminal surface of enterocytes. There was no evidence of villous atrophy despite viral adhesion and colonization (Fig. 2).[22] These findings are strongly indicative of intestinal tropism of SARS coronavirus. With the high viral load in the intestine, it is not difficult to envisage the passage of virus into patients' feces. Peiris *et al.* have reported that the virus can be detected by RT-PCR in the stool samples of all 20 patients with positive nasopharynegeal aspirates at day 10 after onset of symptoms.[6] At day 21, 67% of these initially positive patients still had viral RNA detected in stool samples. An independent study has further shown that virus can be detected by PCR in stool for up to 73 days from symptoms onset in a patient.[22] The long carriage of virus in patients' feces has great implications for transmission of infection and infection control. Though diarrhea is a common manifestation of SARS, many questions remain unanswered. It remains elusive whether the route of transmission (respiratory *versus* fecal-oral) is important in determining the gastrointestinal manifestation

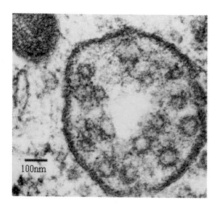 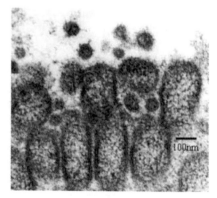

Fig. 2 Ultrastructural appearances of terminal ileum in a patient with SARS. Endoscopic terminal ileal biopsies obtained from a patient with SARS. *Left:* A dilated cytoplasmic vesicle filled with viral particles. Right: Viral particles were detected on the surface micro-villi of the surface enterocyte.

of SARS.[6,24,25] Moreover, further studies are necessary to characterize the mechanism underlying the diarrhea related to SARS-coronavirus infection.

HEMATOLOGICAL FEATURES IN SARS

Hematological features of SARS offer important early clues to the diagnosis of the disease. Initial and progressive lymphopenia (absolute lymphocyte count $<1000/mm^3$) was highly prevalent (98%) among patients suffering from SARS.[23] In fact, the absence of progressive lymphopenia would be rather unusual and alternative diagnoses need to be considered. In most cases, the lymphocyte count was lowest in the second week and started to recover in the third week of illness that coincides with clinical improvement. However, 30% of patients remain lymphopenic at the fifth week of SARS. In addition, both CD4 [on presentation, 286.7 cells/µl (SD 142.2); normal range, 410–1590 cells/µl] and CD8 T-lymphocyte counts [on presentation 242.2 cells/µl (SD 130.8); normal range, 62–559 cells/µl] decrease early in the course of illness. These counts reach their trough in 5–14 days after onset of illness, and then recover gradually. The CD4/CD8 ratio is constant. Notably, the B-lymphocytes are relatively unaffected. It was also found that lower counts of CD4 and CD8 cells actually correlate with adverse clinical outcomes of ICU admission and/or death. Besides, thrombocytopenia (55%) followed by reactive thrombocytosis (49%), and isolated prolonged activated thromboplastin time (63%) are commonly observed. Disseminated intravascular coagulopathy rarely occurs.

LIVER DERANGEMENT IN SARS

Elevated alanine aminotransferase (ALT) levels were frequently reported in SARS patients. Data from recent cohorts showed that 22–56% of patients had elevated ALT at the time of hospital admission.[4] Our recent analysis has shown that 24% of patients had elevation of ALT on admission and up to 69% patients had transient elevation of ALT during the course of illness (Chan, unpublished data). The reason for the liver derangement remains elusive, but evidence of direct hepatotoxic effect by the coronavirus is lacking on autopsy examination. Interestingly, Peiris *et al.* reported that patients with chronic hepatitis B had more severe respiratory disease, despite the fact that patients in that cohort had normal ALT levels and no stigmata of liver cirrhosis on admission.[6]

ATYPICAL MANIFESTATIONS OF SARS

As mentioned earlier, fever >38°C may not be detected on presentation and careful follow-up of the clinical course is necessary. However, some SARS patients may never mount a fever response to *coronavirus* infection as in any other causes of pneumonia. In this regard, elderly SARS patients may have no documented fever even in the presence of progressive pneumonia.[27-30] The WHO/CDC criteria for SARS, when applied to frail older adults-who tend to present with geriatric syndromes of falls, confusion, incontinence, and poor feeding-have their limitations.[27] Instead of a temperature of more than 38°C, a different fever pattern may be observed. Also, patients may not present with respiratory but gastrointestinal symptoms, such as diarrhea, nausea, or vomiting, which, in frail elderly persons, may mimic fecal incontinence and poor feeding. Elders with SARS often have a longer incubation period of 14 to 21 days because of delayed detection and inexact day of contact. This has important clinical implications for diagnosis, contact tracing, duration of surveillance, and infection control measures during high-risk nursing and personal care. The frequent occurrence of concurrent illnesses (e.g. aspiration pneumonia) in old age may also mask the diagnosis of SARS. A retrospective study showed that two-thirds (100 out of 150) of elderly patients (≥65 years old) referred for suspected SARS had alternative diagnosis, compared with only one-third of younger patients. Because the presentations of SARS in the elderly can be nonspecific, a positive contact history may be the first important clue. Thus, a diagnosis of SARS in old age requires a high index of suspicion, knowledge of the presentations of infections in old age, awareness of the age-assessment changes in physical and functional state, alertness to any contact history of SARS, and an updated knowledge of the current prevalence of SARS in the locality.

Apart from senility, diagnosis of SARS is more difficult in the presence of co-morbidities and in immunocompromised patients. Patients who are immunocompromised (e.g. chronic renal failure or in those who were on immunosuppressive therapy, including corticosteroid) may present with respiratory illness and pneumonia without fever.[28,29] Symptoms may be vague and the typical triphasic pattern could be absent. Moreover, plain chest radiographs are difficult to interpret in patients with pre-existing chronic pulmonary diseases (e.g. pulmonary fibrosis), and in the presence of pulmonary edema (e.g. congestive heart failure).

On the other hand, radiological features of SARS may mimic some of these conditions.

Patients with SARS could present with unrelated medical or even surgical conditions prior to the ultimate manifestations of SARS. There are reports of SARS patients presenting with as acute pulmonary edema, exacerbation of chronic obstructive airway disease, influenza, bacteremia, acute abdomen and even hip fracture.[29–33] These "hidden" SARS patients are the most challenging to the infection control and healthcare systems. Unrecognized cases of SARS have been implicated in recent outbreaks in Singapore, Taiwan, and Toronto. Thus, a high index of suspicion, the availability of a sensitive and specific virological testing, and the judicious use of high resolution CT scan of thorax (HRCT) may be useful in the early diagnosis of SARS.[18] The need for a rapid and reliable diagnostic test cannot be over-emphasized.

SARS can rarely present as hemorrhagic fever-like illness. There is report of patients presenting with early features of disseminated intravascular coagulopathy, including thrombocytopenia, prolonged activated thromboplastin time and elevated D-dimer levels. Radiological abnormalities developed later in the course of the illness.[34]

CONCLUSIONS

Early manifestation of SARS is characterized by non-specific symptoms and signs. With the increased recognition of atypical presentation of SARS, accurate and prompt diagnosis of SARS based on clinical grounds alone may be difficult. Careful history taking, contact tracing, follow up of symptom evolution, and serial monitoring of chest radiographs are essential in the early diagnosis of SARS, which is the best way in containing the further spread of the infection.[35] The need for a rapid diagnostic test with high sensitivity and specificity cannot be overemphasized.

REFERENCES

1. Drosten C, Gunther S, Preiser W, *et al.* Identification of a novel coronavirus in patients with severe acute respiratory syndrome. *N Engl J Med* 2003;**348**:1967–76.

2. WHO. Severe acute respiratory syndrome (SARS). http://www.who.int/csr/media/sars.

3. CDC. Updated interim surveillance case definition for severe acute respiratory syndrome (SARS). http://www.cdc.gov/ncidod/sars/casedefinition.

4. Lee N, Hui D, Wu A, *et al.* A major outbreak of severe acute respiratory syndrome in Hong Kong. *N Engl J Med* 2003;**348**:1986–94.

5. Booth CM, Matukas LM, Tomlinson GA, *et al.* Clinical features and short-term outcomes of 144 patients with SARS in the greater Toronto area. *JAMA* 2003;**289**:2801–9.

6. Peiris JS, Chu CM, Cheng VC, *et al.* Clinical progression and viral load in a community outbreak of coronavirus-associated SARS pneumonia: A prospective study. *Lancet* 2003;**361**:1767–72.

7. Wu W, Wang J, Liu P, *et al.* A hospital outbreak of severe acute respiratory syndrome in GuangZhou, China. *Chin Med J* (Engl) 2003;**116**:811–8.

8. Hsu LY, Lee CC, Green JA, *et al.* Severe acute respiratory syndrome (SARS) in Singapore: Clinical features of index patient and initial contacts. *Emerg Infect Dis* 2003;**9**:713–7.

9. Donnelly CA, Ghani AC, Leung GM, *et al.* Epidemiological determinants of spread of causal agent of severe acute respiratory syndrome in Hong Kong. *Lancet* 2003;**361**:1761–6.

10. Rainer TH, Cameron PA, Smith D, *et al.* Evaluation of WHO criteria for identifying patients with severe acute respiratory syndrome out of hospital: Prospective observational study. *BMJ* 2003;**326**:1354–8.

11. Wong GWK, Hui DSC. Severe acute respiratory syndrome (SARS): Epidemiology, diagnosis and management. *Thorax* 2003;**58**:558–60.

12. David SC Hui, Joseph JY Sung. Severe acute respiratory syndrome. *Chest* 2003;**124**:12–15.

13. Wong KT, Antonio GE, Jui D, *et al.* Severe acute respiratory syndrome: Radiographic appearances and pattern of progression in 138 patients. *Radiology* 2003;**228**:401–6.

14. So L, Lau A, Yam L, *et al.* Development of a standard treatment protocol for severe acute respiratory syndrome. *Lancet* 2003;**361**:1615–6.

15. Ho JC, Ooi GC, Mok TY, *et al.* High dose pulse versus non-pulse corticosteroid regimens in severe acute respiratory syndrome. *Am J Respir Crit Care Med* 2003;**168**:1449–56.

16. Lew TW, Kwek TK, Tai D, *et al.* Acute respiratory distress syndrome in critically ill patients with severe acute respiratory syndrome. *JAMA* 2003;**290**:374–80.

17. Fowler RA, Lapinsky SE, Hallett D, *et al.* Toronto SARS critical care group. Critically ill patients with severe acute respiratory syndrome. *JAMA* 2003;**290**:367–73.

18. Wong KT, Antonio GE, Hui D, *et al.* Thin-section CT of severe acute respiratory syndrome: Evaluation of 73 patients exposed to or with the disease. *Radiology* 2003;**228**:395–400.

19. Nicholls JM, Poon LL, Lee KC, *et al.* Lung pathology of fatal severe acute respiratory syndrome *Lancet* 2003;**361**:1773–8.

20. Mazzulli T, Farcas GA, Poutanen SM, *et al.* Severe acute respiratory syndrome-associated coronavirus in lung tissue. *Emerg Infect Dis* 2004;**10**:20–24.

21. Tsui PT, Kwok ML, Yuen H, Lai ST. Severe acute respiratory syndrome: Clinical outcome and prognostic correlates. *Emerg Infect Dis* 2003;**9**:1064–9.

22. Leung WK, To KF, Chan PKS, *et al.* Enteric manifestation of severe acute respiratory syndrome (SARS) — Associated coronavirus infection. *Gastroenterology* 2003;**125**:1011–7.

23. Hon K, Li AM, Cheng F, Leung TF, NG PC. Personal view of SARS: Confusing definition, confusing diagnoses. *Lancet* 2003;**361**:1984–5.

24. Government of Hong Kong Special Administrative Region, Department of Health. Outbreak of severe acute respiratory syndrome (SARS) at Amoy Gardens, Kowloon Bay, Hong Kong. http://www.info.gov.hk/info/ap/pdf/amoy_e.pdf

25. Riley S, Fraser C, Donnelly CA, *et al.* Transmission dynamics of the etiological agent of SARS in Hong Kong: Impact of public health interventions. *Science* 2003;**300**:1961–6.

26. Wong R, Wu A, To KF, *et al.* Haematological manifestations in patients with severe acute respiratory syndrome: Retrospective analysis. *BMJ* 2003;**326**:1358–62.

27. Kong TK, Dai DLK, Leung MF. Severe acute respiratory syndrome in elders. *JAGS* 2003;**S1**:1182.

28. Sampathkumar P, Temesgen Z, Smith TF, Thompson RL. SARS: Epidemiology, clinical presentation, management, and infection control measures. *Mayo Clin Proc* 2003;**78**:882–90.

29. Fisher DA, Lim TK, Lim YT, Singh KS, Tambyah PA. Atypical presentations of SARS. Lancet 2003;**361**:1740.

30. Wong KC, Leung KS, Hui M. Severe acute respiratory syndrome (SARS) in a geriatric patient with a hip fracture. *Bone Joint Surg* 2003 (In press).

31. CDC. Severe acute respiratory syndrome — Singapore, 2003. *MMWR* 2003;**52**:405–11. http://www.cdc.gov/mmwr/preview/mmwrhtml/mm5218a1.htm

32. CDC. Cluster of severe acute respiratory syndrome cases among protected health care workers — Toronto, April 2003. *MMWR* 2003;**52**:433–6. http://www.cdc.gov/mmwr/preview/mmwrhtml/mm5219a1.htm

33. CDC. Severe acute respiratory syndrome — Taiwan, 2003. *MMWR* 2003;**52**:461–66. http://www.cdc.gov/mmwr/preview/mmwrhtml/mm5220a1.htm

34. Wu EB, Sung JY. Hemorrhagic-like-fever changes and a normal chest radiograph in a doctor of SARS. *Lancet* 2003;**361**:1520.

35. Fisher DA, Chew MHL, Lim YT, Tambyah PA. Preventing local transmission of SARS: Lessons from Singapore. *MJA* 2003;**178**:555–58.

5

Clinical Diagnosis

David SC Hui

INTRODUCTION

SARS is described as a new clinical entity during the March 2003 outbreak in Hong Kong, Hanoi and Singapore. The name SARS and its case definition was first introduced by the World Health Organization on 15 March 2003.[1] Subsequently, the Center of Diseases Control in the US has issued a separate set of guidelines and case definitions. During the recent SARS epidemic and before the identification of SARS-CoV, the diagnosis of SARS depended on recognition of certain clinical, laboratory and radiological features in addition to identification of any epidemiological linkage to an index case.

CLINICAL, LABORATORY AND RADIOLOGICAL FEATURES

The incubation period of SARS is generally between 2 and 10 days with a mean of 6.4 days, and the time interval from onset of clinical symptoms to hospital admission is between 3 and 5 days.[2] The frequency of presentation of clinical features from several case series is as summarized in Table 1. The

Table 1 Clinical Features of SARS on Presentation[3-5]

Symptoms	% of Patients with Symptoms
Persistent fever >38°C	99–100
Non-productive cough	57–75
Myalgia	45–61
Chills/rigor	15–73
Headache	20–56
Dyspnea	40–42
Malaise	31–45
Nausea and vomiting	20–35
Diarrhea	20–25
Sore throat	13–25
Dizziness	4.2–43
Sputum production	4.9–29
Rhinorrhea	2.1–23
Arthralgia	10.4

major clinical features include persistent fever, chills/rigor, myalgia, malaise, dry cough, headache and dyspnea. Less common symptoms include sputum production, sore throat, coryza, dizziness, nausea, vomiting, and diarrhea.[3-5] Watery diarrhea was reported in 73% of a group of patients one week down the clinical course in a community outbreak linked to a faulty sewage system in Hong Kong, presumably due to involvement of the gastrointestinal tract via the fecal oral route.[6] Nevertheless, these clinical symptoms are rather non-specific and may be due to influenza or other causes of atypical pneumonia, such as mycoplasma, chlamydia, and legionella. Older subjects may present with deterioration in general condition, poor feeding, fall/fracture,[7] and in some cases, delirium, without the typical febrile response.[7,8] Physical examination of patients with SARS may reveal fever, tachypnea, tachycardia and inspiratory crackles at the lung bases in some cases.[3-5]

Laboratory features such as lymphopenia, features of low grade disseminated intravascular coagulation (thrombocytopenia, prolonged activated partial thromboplastin time, elevated D-Dimer), elevated lactate dehydrogenase (LDH) (reflecting lung injury), and creatinine kinase (reflecting myositis) are commonly observed in SARS. These laboratory abnormalities, together with the clinical features, may help in the clinical diagnosis of SARS.[3-6] The CD4 and CD8 T lymphocyte counts fall early in the course of SARS, whereas low counts of CD4 and CD8 at presentation are associated with adverse outcome.[9]

The clinical course of SARS appears to follow a typical pattern in many cases: Phase 1 (viral replication) is associated with an increasing viral load and clinically characterized by fever, myalgia, and other systemic symptoms that generally improve after a few days. Phase 2 (immunopathological damage) is characterized by recurrence of fever, oxygen desaturation, radiological progression of pneumonia with decrease in viral load. The majority of patients will improve with a combination of ribavirin and intravenous steroid therapy, but 20% of patients may progress to acute respiratory distress syndrome (ARDS), necessitating ventilatory support.[6] Compared with adults and teenagers, SARS seems to run a less aggressive clinical course in younger children, and none of the children aged below 13 years required supplementary oxygen in a case series.[10]

Previous studies have shown that there are no specific radiographic features that can reliably distinguish bacterial from non-bacterial causes of pneumonia.[11] The radiographic appearances of SARS, indeed, share common features with other causes of pneumonia. At onset of fever, about 80% of the patients with SARS have abnormal chest radiographs, all of which showing air-space consolidation. All the patients will eventually develop lung opacities during the course of the disease. The opacities occupy a peripheral or mixed peripheral and axial location in 88% of cases.[12] The more distinctive radiographic features of SARS are the predominant involvement of lung periphery and the lower zone, and the absence of cavitation, hilar lymphadenopathy or pleural effusion.[3,12] It is common to see radiographic progression from unilateral focal air-space opacity to either multi-focal or bilateral involvement during the second week of the disease, followed by radiographic improvement with intravenous steroid treatment.[3,12] Despite the use of low volume and low pressure during mechanical ventilation, the incidence of barotrauma seems higher than expected. In a case series, 12% of patients developed spontaneous pneumo-mediastinum and 20% of patients developed evidence of ARDS over a period of 3 weeks.[6] Chest radiographs and CT scans have not demonstrated excessive hyperinflation or bullous lung disease,[13] and the high incidence of barotraumas is likely related to poor lung compliance.

Among the 20% of cases with initially unremarkable chest radiographs, high resolution CT of the thorax is useful in detecting parenchymal opacities. Common findings include ground-glass opacification, sometimes with consolidation, and interlobular septal and intralobular interstitial thickening, with predominantly a peripheral and lower lobe involvement. The characteristic peripheral alveolar opacities closely resemble those found in bronchiolitis obliterans organizing pneumonia.[3,13]

DIAGNOSTIC CRITERIA OF SARS

Both the WHO and the CDC have issued updated case definitions for SARS during the outbreak. A suspected case has been defined by the WHO (revised 1 May 2003)[14] as a person presenting (after 1 November 2002) with:

- Fever >38°C, plus
- Cough or difficulty breathing, plus
- Either close contact with a person who is a suspect or probable case of SARS and/or history of travel or residence in an area with recent local transmission of SARS within 10 days of onset of symptoms.

Patients with an unexplained fatal acute respiratory illness who fit the above epidemiologic criteria, but on whom no autopsy has been performed, are also classified as suspected cases. A probable case is defined as:

- A suspected case with radiographic findings of pneumonia or acute respiratory distress syndrome (ARDS), or
- A suspected case positive for SAR CoV in one or more laboratory assays, or
- A suspected case with autopsy evidence of ARDS with unknown cause.

The WHO definitions have been established to assist in the definition of hospital cases. The reason for retaining the clinical and epidemiological basis for the case definitions is that there is as yet no validated, widely and consistently available rapid test for SARS CoV infection. The WHO definitions have recently been evaluated in the context of screening patients before admission to hospital.[15] In the early stages of SARS, the main discriminating features are fever, chills, malaise, myalgia, rigors rather than cough and breathing difficulty. Documented fever (>38°C) may not occur in the early stages in some cases, and radiological evidence of pneumonic changes often precedes fever. The WHO case definitions for suspected SARS have a low sensitivity of 26% and a negative predictive value of 85% for detecting SARS in patients who have not been admitted to hospital.[15] The WHO has recently revised the case definitions in the post-outbreak period on 14 August 2003, with inclusion of radiographic and laboratory findings for public health purposes (Table 2).[16]

The CDC case definitions of SARS are based on clinical, epidemiologic, and laboratory criteria (Table 3).[17] The CDC criteria differ from those of the WHO in that respiratory symptoms for severe cases are included. The case definitions and exclusion criteria have been revised to allow exclusion of cases with a convalescent phase serum sample,

---

Table 2 WHO Case Definitions of SARS in the Post-outbreak Period[16]

Clinical case definition of SARS:
A person with a history of:
Fever $\geq 38°C$
AND one or more symptoms of lower respiratory tract illness (cough, difficulty in breathing, shortness of breath)
AND
Radiographic evidence of lung infiltrates consistent with pneumonia or (respiratory distress syndrome) RDS **OR** autopsy findings consistent with the pathology of pneumonia or RDS without an identifiable cause.
AND
No alternative diagnosis can fully explain the illness.

Laboratory case definition of SARS:
A person with symptoms and signs that are clinically suggestive of SARS AND with positive laboratory findings for SARS CoV based on one or more of the following diagnostic criteria:

(a) PCR positive for SARS CoV
   PCR positive using a validated method from:
   • At least 2 different clinical specimens (e.g. nasopharyngeal aspirate or stool), OR
   • The same clinical specimen collected on 2 or more occasions during the course of the illness (e.g. sequential nasopharyngeal aspirates), OR
   • Two different assays or repeat PCR using a new RNA extract from the original clinical sample on each occasion of testing.
(b) Seroconversion by ELISA or IFA
   • Negative antibody test on acute serum followed by positive antibody test on convalescent phase serum tested in parallel, OR
   • Fourfold or greater rise in antibody titre between acute and convalescent phase sera tested in parallel.
(c) Virus isolation
   Isolation in cell culture of SARS CoV from any specimen AND PCR confirmation using a validated method.

Table 3 CDC Updated Interim Case Definition for SARS[17]

Clinical Criteria:
(a)   Asymptomatic or mild respiratory illness.
(b)   Moderate respiratory illness (temp >100.4°F or 38°C) and at least one respiratory feature (cough, dyspnea, difficulty in breathing, or hypoxia).
(c)   Severe respiratory illness (features of b and radiographic evidence of pneumonia, or respiratory distress syndrome, or autopsy findings consistent with pneumonia, or respiratory distress syndrome without an identifiable cause).

Epidemiologic Criteria:
Travel (including transit in an airport) within 10 days of onset of symptoms to an area with current or recently documented or suspected community transmission of SARS, or Close contact within 10 days of onset of symptoms with a person known or suspected to have SARS infection.

Laboratory Criteria:
(a)   Confirmed:
      Detection of antibody to SARS-CoV in specimens obtained during acute illness or 21 days after illness onset, or
      Detection of SARS-CoV RNA by reverse-transcriptase polymerase chain reaction (RT-PCR), confirmed by a second PCR assay, by using a second aliquot of the specimen and a different set of PCR primers, or
      Isolation of SARS-CoV.
(b)   Negative:
      Absence of antibody to SARS CoV in a convalescent phase sample obtained >28 days after onset of symptoms.
(c)   Undetermined: Laboratory test either not performed or incomplete.

Case Classification:
A case of *probable SARS* is defined as having met the clinical criteria for *severe* respiratory illness of unknown aetiology and epidemiologic criteria for exposure, laboratory criteria confirmed or undetermined.
A case of *suspect SARS* is defined as having met the clinical criteria for *moderate* respiratory illness of unknown aetiology, and epidemiologic criteria for exposure, laboratory criteria confirmed or undetermined.

Exclusion Criteria:
A case may be excluded as a suspect or probable SARS case if:
(a)   An alternative diagnosis can fully explain the illness.
(b)   The case has a convalescent phase serum sample (i.e. obtained >28 days after onset of symptoms) for which is negative for antibody to SARS-CoV.
(c)   The case was reported on the basis of contact with an index case that was subsequently excluded as a case of SARS, provided other possible epidemiologic exposure criteria are not present.

collected more than 28 days after symptom onset, that is, negative for antibody to SARS-CoV.

Obviously, a clinical diagnosis of SARS based on clinical and radiographic features has its pitfalls. The non-discriminating lower respiratory tract symptoms,[15] non-specific radiographic features,[12] and atypical presentations[7,8] especially in the elderly, may pose greater difficulties in the management of SARS. Thus, a rapid, reliable and early diagnostic test is urgently needed to facilitate management and control of the spread of the infection.

CONCLUSION

In conclusion, with the recent onset of the SARS epidemic worldwide, research in the development of diagnostic tests is urgently needed. The availability of the genome sequence of the SARS CoV[18-20] will hopefully facilitate efforts to develop new and rapid diagnostic tests. The WHO[1,14] and CDC[17] case definitions of SARS during the outbreak period, are greatly dependent on epidemiological linkage to increase the specificity of the diagnostic criteria. Nevertheless, in the post-epidemic period, epidemiological links to cases of SARS as well as to areas reporting recent local transmissions, are no longer useful in defining incident cases.[16] The clinical and laboratory features of SARS are non-specific and may be indistinguishable from other cases of atypical pneumonia. However, the constellation of compatible clinical and laboratory findings, together with the radiological features, especially on HRCT, and the lack of clinical response to broad-spectrum antibiotics, should quickly arouse our suspicion of SARS. Until rapid diagnostic tests with a high rate of early detection become readily available, the diagnosis of SARS will remain a clinical decision, with exclusion of other causes of atypical pneumonia, in the early stages.

REFERENCES

1. World Health Organization. Case definitions for surveillance of severe acute respiratory syndrome (SARS) from: http://www.who.int/csr/sars/casedefinition/en. (accessed April 10, 2003).

2. Donnelly CA, Ghani AV, Leung GM, *et al.* Epidemiological determinants of spread of causal agent of severe acute respiratory syndrome in Hong Kong. *Lancet* 2003;**361**:1761–6.

3. Lee N, Hui DS, Wu A, *et al.* A major outbreak of severe acute respiratory syndrome in Hong Kong. *N Engl J Med* 2003;**348**:1986–94.

4. Hsu LY, Lee CC, Green JA, *et al.* Severe acute respiratory syndrome in Singapore: Clinical features of index patient and initial contacts. *Emerg Infect Dis* 2003;**9**:713–7.

5. Booth CM, Matukas LM, Tomlinson GA, *et al.* Clinical features and short-term outcomes of 144 patients with SARS in the greater Toronto area. *JAMA* 2003;**289**:2801–9.

6. Peiris JS, Chu CM, Cheng VC, *et al.* Clinical progression and viral load in a community outbreak of coronavirus-associated SARS pneumonia: A prospective study. *Lancet* 2003;**361**:1767–72.

7. Wong KC, Leung KS, Hui M. Severe acute respiratory syndrome (SARS) in a geriatric patient with a hip fracture. A case report. *J Bone Joint Surg Am* 2003;**85A**:1339–42.

8. Fisher DA, Lim TK, Lim YT, *et al.* Atypical presentations of SARS. *Lancet* 2003;**361**:1740.

9. Wong RS, Wu A, To KF, *et al.* Haematological manifestations in patients with severe acute respiratory syndrome: Retrospective analysis. *Brit Med J* 2003;**326**:1358–62.

10. Hon KL, Leung CW, Cheng WT, *et al.* Clinical presentations and outcome of severe acute respiratory syndrome in children. *Lancet* 2003;**361**:1701–3.

11. Marrie TJ. Community acquired pneumonia. *Clin Infect Dis* 1994;**18**:501–13.

12. Wong KT, Antonio GE, Hui DS, *et al.* Radiographic appearances and pattern of progression of severe acute respiratory syndrome (SARS): A study of 138 patients. *Radiology* 2003;**228**:401–6.

13. Wong KT, Antonio GE, Hui DS, *et al.* Thin-section CT of severe acute respiratory syndrome: Evaluation of 73 patients exposed to or with the disease. *Radiology* 2003;**228**:395–400.

14. World Health Organization. Case definitions for surveillance of severe acute respiratory syndrome (SARS): http://www.who.int/csr/sars/csedefinition/en/print.html. (accessed July 10, 2003).

15. Rainer TH, Cameron PA, Smit D, *et al.* Evaluation of WHO criteria for identifying patients with severe acute respiratory syndrome out of hospital: Prospective observational study. *Brit Med J* 2003;**326**:1354–8.

16. World Health Organization. Alert, verification and public health management of SARS in the post outbreak period: http://www.who.int/csr/sars/postoutbreak/en/print.html. (accessed Aug 17, 2003).

17. CDC. Updated interim US case definition for severe acute respiratory syndrome (SARS) (July 10, 2003): http://www.cdc.gov/ncidod/sars/pdf/sars-casedefinition.pdf (accessed July 29, 2003).

18. Rota PA, Oberste MS, Monroe SS, *et al.* Characterization of a novel coronavirus associated with severe acute respiratory syndrome. *Science* 2003;**300**:1394–9.

19. Marra MA, Jones SJ, Astell CR, *et al.* The genome sequence of the SARS-associated coronavirus. *Science* 2003;**300**:1399–404.

20. Ruan YJ, Wei CL, Ee LA, *et al.* Comparative full-length genome sequence analysis of 14 SARS coronavirus isolates and common mutations associated with putative origins of infection. *Lancet* 2003;**361**:1779–85.

6

Laboratory Diagnosis

Enders KO Ng, YM Dennis Lo

INTRODUCTION

Despite the subsidence of the severe acute respiratory syndrome (SARS) epidemic in many parts of the world, many authorities have warned of the possible re-emergence of this highly infectious disease. The Centers for Disease Control and Prevention (CDC) and the World Health Organization (WHO) have repeatedly emphasized the need for developing better diagnostic tests for SARS.

After the etiologic agent of SARS was identified as the SARS-coronavirus (SARS-CoV),[1–6] various diagnostic tests have been developed by different research groups around the world. However, the progress in the development of sensitive and early diagnostic tests for SARS has been slower than originally expected. Most of the diagnostic tests are not sensitive enough for detection during the early phase of the disease. For instance, the use of nasopharyngeal aspirates has a sensitivity of only 32% on day 3 of the disease.[7] This severe limitation has restricted our ability to identify patients in a prompt manner and to institute isolation and treatment.

In this chapter, some of the laboratory diagnostic approaches for SARS-coronavirus infection are discussed. In addition, several promising new technologies will be reviewed.

DIAGNOSTIC APPROACHES

Viral Culture

The isolation of an infectious virus can be achieved by inoculating patient specimens, such as respiratory secretions, urine, blood or stool with suitable cell lines (e.g. Vero cells). During incubation, if cytopathic effect is seen on cell cultures, viruses will be isolated and further tests, such as electron microscopy, can be used to identify the virus. Virus isolation from cell culture provides a means to demonstrate the presence of a living virus. Previous studies have reported the successful culture of SARS-CoV from various specimen types, including sputum, nasal swab, throat wash, kidney and lung biopsy.[1-4] This approach was one of the original means used for isolating and identifying the novel coronavirus from SARS patients. Recently, the positivity of virus culture from various specimen types was examined. Respiratory specimens have 14–66% positivity during the first week of illness, dropping to 5–14% at day 21. Urine and stool specimens have a very low positive rate (1–2%) during the first three weeks of illness (unpublished data from Prof. Paul Chan, Department of Microbiology, The Chinese University of Hong Kong). Despite the usefulness of this test, this method requires cell culturing which is time-consuming and has to be conducted in a laboratory with proper containment facilities. Furthermore, negative cytopathic results do not always exclude the presence of SARS-CoV in the sample tested.

ANTIBODY DETECTION BY SEROLOGY

Various methods can be used to detect the antibodies generated in response to SARS-CoV infection. The most common methodology is the immunofluorescence assay (IFA) in which antibodies from the serum of patients bind to SARS-CoV-infected cells fixed on a microscope slide.[1,2,7] The antibody-antigen complexes are in turn detected by fluorescence-labeled secondary antibodies under a fluorescence microscope. In addition to IFA, other detection methods, such as enzyme-linked immunosorbent assay (ELISA), are also becoming available.[8]

In antibody testing, a patient with a positive result (seroconversion from negative to positive or a 4-fold increase in antibody titre) indicates previous SARS-CoV infection. In previous studies, it has been reported that about 50% of SARS patients had IgG seroconversion at around 15 days after symptoms onset.[7] At a mean of 20 days, 93% of patients had evidence of IgG seroconversion. Recently, another laboratory studied the profile of IgM and IgG responses to SARS-CoV infection. The data demonstrated that 100% of 20 SARS patients were IgG-positive after 21 days and continued to have high IgG titres up to three months after symptoms onset.[8] Conversely, the IgM titre peaked during the acute or early convalescent phase and then declined to undetectable levels by the end of week 12.[8] Although antibody detection provides a highly sensitive and specific diagnosis of SARS-CoV infection, it is not suitable for early diagnosis because positive results are normally generated relatively late in the course of the illness.

PCR-BASED DIAGNOSTIC TESTS

Based on the publicly released full genomic sequences of SARS-CoV,[9–11] various molecular detection methods have been developed. Most of molecular tests developed are based on reverse transcriptase polymerase chain reaction (RT–PCR), in which viral RNA is reverse-transcribed into DNA and then different regions of the SARS-CoV genome are specifically amplified by PCR. Several RT–PCR protocols developed by members of the WHO laboratory network are available on the WHO website (http://www.who.int/csr/sars/primers/en/).

Conventional RT–PCR approaches are normally qualitative in nature and require time-consuming and contamination-prone post-PCR analysis. Real-time quantitative RT–PCR has overcome many of these shortcomings and has been increasingly adopted by various laboratories.[2,12–14] This technique is based on the performance of RT–PCR in the presence of a dual-labeled fluorescent probe, which allows the fluorescence signals to be recorded and analyzed during PCR cycling. This methodology runs as a closed-tube system and post-amplification manipulation can be eliminated. Thus, it reduces the risk of contamination and minimizes hands-on time. The entire amplification process requires only three hours and allows such technology to be used for high-throughput application.

PREVENTION OF CONTAMINATION

Due to the high sensitivity of PCR-based approaches, strict precautions should be applied to prevent the RT–PCR assay from contamination.[15] These precautions include:

1. Aerosol-resistant pipette tips should be used for all liquid handling.
2. Separate areas should be used for the RNA extraction step, the setting up of amplification reactions, the addition of template and the carrying out of amplification reactions.
3. Instead of using a two-step RT–PCR approach, a one-step RT–PCR, incorporating both the reverse transcription and PCR steps in a single tube, should be used to reduce both hands-on time and the risk of contamination.
4. Real-time PCR approaches obviate the need for post-PCR processing and further reduce the risk of contamination.
5. The assay should include a further level of anti-contamination measure in the form of pre-amplification treatment, using uracil N-glycosylase which destroys uracil containing PCR products.[16]
6. Multiple negative water blanks should be included in every analysis so as to eliminate the possibility of reagent contamination.

RT–PCR USING RESPIRATORY SECRETIONS, URINE OR STOOL SAMPLES

Initially, molecular testing for SARS has mainly been focused on RT–PCR analysis of nasopharyngeal aspirates, urine and stools.[7,12] In one of the previous studies, SARS-CoV RNA was detected in 32% of nasopharyngeal aspirates from SARS patients studied at a mean of 3.2 days after symptom onset.[7] The detection rate increased to 68% at day 14. In the same study, SARS-CoV RNA was detected in 97% of stool samples collected at a mean of 14.2 days after symptom onset. Similarly, viral RNA was detected in 42% of urine samples collected from the SARS patients at a mean of 15.2 days after onset.[7] Despite the high sensitivity of stool sample testing, early detection of SARS-CoV still suffers from a lack of sensitivity.

RT–PCR USING PLASMA SAMPLE

Although most of the assays have been predominantly focused on RNA extracted from nasopharyngeal aspirates, urine and stools, the quantitative interpretation of these data is difficult due to the inability to standardize such data as a result of the influence of numerous factors, such as sampling technique for nasopharyngeal aspirates, urine volume, variations of bowel transit time (e.g. during diarrhea), or stool consistency. On the other hand, plasma/serum-based assays may allow the precise and standardized quantitative expression of viral loads, thus enabling the assessment of disease severity and prognosis. Detection of viral nucleic acids in plasma/serum has been well-established for viral load studies for numerous other viruses.[17,18] At the beginning of the SARS outbreak, there has been a single report showing the relatively low sensitivity of detecting SARS-CoV RNA in plasma using an ultracentrifugation-based approach, with low concentrations of SARS-CoV detected in the plasma of a patient 9 days after disease onset.[2] Subsequently, together with the improvement of viral RNA extraction in which plasma or serum required no ultracentrifugation, two real-time quantitative RT–PCR assays, one towards the polymerase region and the other towards the nucleocapsid region of the virus genome, were developed for measuring the concentration of SARS-CoV RNA in serum/plasma samples from SARS patients.[13,14] In these assays, the absolute calibration curves are constructed by serial dilutions of high performance liquid chromatography (HPLC)-purified single stranded synthetic DNA oligonucleotides specifying the studied amplicons (see Fig. 1). Previous studies have shown that such single stranded oligonucleotides reliably mimic the products of the reverse transcription step and produce calibration curves that are identical to those obtained using T7-transcribed RNA.[19,20] The use of such calibration methodology does offer advantages. For example, the commercial availability of synthetic oligonucleotides significantly simplifies the process of obtaining a calibration curve as compared with the labour-intensive preparation of calibration curve which involves amplicon subcloning and *in vitro* transcription.

The sensitivities of the amplification steps of these assays are sufficient to detect five copies of the targets in the reaction mixtures, corresponding to 74 copies/mL of plasma/serum. The coefficients of variation for the polymerase and nucleocapsid amplification systems are 16.4% at 280 copies/mL and 14.9% at 320 copies/mL, respectively.[13] Using these

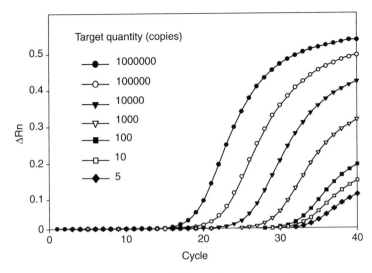

Fig. 1 Detection of SARS-CoV RNA by real-time quantitative RT–PCR for the polymerase region of the viral genome. An amplification plot of ΔRn, which is the fluorescence intensity over the background (Y-axis) against the PCR cycle number (X-axis). Each plot corresponds to a particular input synthetic DNA oligonucleotide target quantity marked by a corresponding symbol.

RT–PCR assays, SARS-CoV RNA was detected in 75% to 78% of plasma/serum samples from SARS patients during the first week of illness.[13] The detection rate dropped to 42% at day 14 after fever onset. Overall, the sensitivities of current diagnostic tests for SARS-CoV is listed in Table 1.

With regard to prognostic implication, median concentrations of serum SARS-CoV RNA in patients who required ICU admission during the course of hospitalization were significantly higher than those who did not require intensive care.[13] (see Fig. 2). These data show that serum SARS-CoV measurement is a prognostic marker which can be used even on the first day of hospital admission. The exact biological explanation for the observed relationship between serum SARS-CoV concentration and prognosis is unclear at present. Possible explanations include a direct pathological effect due to the presence of numerous infectious virions which could infect and destroy susceptible cells within the body; or an indirect effect due to the activation of a potentially damaging immune reaction. The elucidation of these possibilities would require future research.

Table 1 Summary of the Sensitivities and Specificities of Currently Available Diagnostic Tests for SARS-CoV

Detection Method	Sensitivity			Specificity
	Day 1	**Day 15**	**Day 21**	
Virus culture				
NPA	18% (61/341)*	14% (15/105)*	0% (0/7)*	ND
Stool	0% (0/22)*	2.4% (1/42)*	0% (0/80)*	ND
Urine	0% (0/111)*	0% (0/92)*	2% (1/50)*	ND
RT–PCR				
Plasma/serum	77% (27/35)[13]	42% (5/12)[13]	ND	100%[13]
NPA	32% (24/75)[7]	68% (51/75)[7]	50% (4/8)*	98%[7]
Stool	33% (7/21)*	97% (65/67)[7]	71% (47/66)*	ND
Urine	2.7% (2/75)*	42% (31/74)[7]	10% (4/39)*	ND
Serology	0%	10%	93–100%[7,8]	ND

ND: Not done
References in superscripts.
*Unpublished data from Prof. Paul Chan.

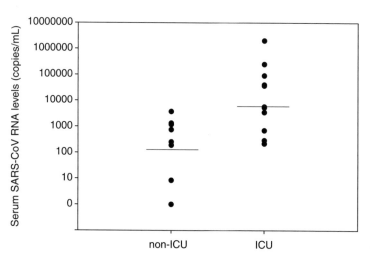

Fig. 2 Serum SARS-CoV RNA levels in SARS patients on the day of hospital admission. Dot plot of SARS-CoV RNA levels (common logarithmic scale) in sera of SARS patients requiring and not requiring ICU admission. Real-time quantitative RT–PCR assays towards the polymerase region of the SARS-CoV genome was used for quantification. The horizontal lines denote the medians.

Although most of the reports were focused on adult SARS patients, recent reports revealed that the clinical course of pediatric SARS patients was less severe in comparison with adult SARS patients.[21,22] On the whole, the outcomes of pediatric SARS patients were favorable. SARS-CoV RNA has recently been shown to be detectable in the plasma samples of pediatric patients during different stages of SARS with drug treatment (see Fig. 3).[14] No significant difference in plasma SARS-CoV viral load has been observed between pediatric and adult SARS patients taken within the first week of admission and at day 7 after fever onset.[14] Overall, viremia appears to be a consistent feature in both pediatric and adult SARS patients.

The relatively high detection of SARS-CoV in plasma and serum during the first week of illness, suggests that plasma/serum-based RT–PCR should be incorporated into the routine diagnostic workup of suspected or confirmed SARS patients both in adult and pediatric populations. The discovery of detectable concentrations of SARS-CoV RNA in the plasma and serum opens up numerous interesting research opportunities. For example, this approach can be used to monitor the effect or lack of effects of anti-viral agents. As a second example, steroids have been used by many groups during the treatment of SARS patients.[22,23] It would be interesting to investigate if high dose steroid treatment might be associated with a prolongation of the duration of viremia. Also, it would be valuable to explore the potential damaging effect of giving steroids at a time when the viral load is still relatively high. We are aware that many of these questions might not be answerable with retrospectively collected samples. Nonetheless, the development of animal models[5,6] might allow the testing of some of these hypotheses in a controled manner.

OTHER APPROACHES

Besides PCR-based detection method, other nucleic acid amplification technologies have opened new avenues for SARS-CoV diagnosis. Most of the amplification technologies amplify target nucleic acids to a similar magnitude, with detection limit of less than 10 copies, but require either a precision instrument for amplification or an elaborate method for detection of the amplified products. A recent method, termed loop-mediated isothermal amplification (LAMP), has been developed which can amplify a few copies of target up to 10 billion-fold in less than half an hour under

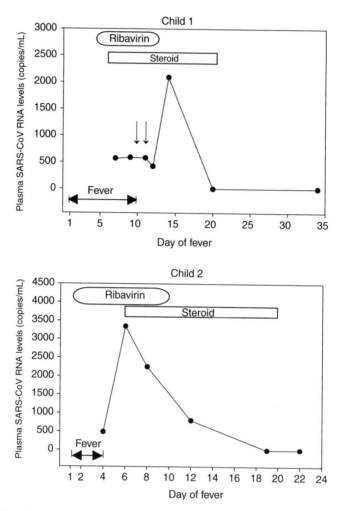

Fig. 3 Serial analysis of plasma SARS-CoV RNA levels in pediatric SARS patients. Plots of plasma SARS-CoV RNA levels (*Y*-axis) against time after the onset of fever (day 1 refers the day of fever onset) (*X*-axis). The duration of fever and the periods of steroid and ribavirin treatment are indicated for each case. The arrows in patient 1 indicate the time of intravenous methylprednisolone treatment.

isothermal conditions and with high specificity.[24] Recently, this new amplification technology has been applied to SARS-CoV detection (http://loopamp.eiken.co.jp) and might provide a rapid and sensitive SARS diagnostic test for small laboratories without suitable instrumentation for real-time quantitative PCR assay.

Furthermore, a technique being used for molecular screening, such as the DNA chip technology (DNA microarray), has been developed and manufactured by a company for rapid re-sequencing of different isolates of the SARS-CoV for investigation of the possible relationship between genomic variations and spread of the SARS-CoV and its virulence (http://www.affymetrix.com). By comparing patient outcome with the pathogen subtypes, researchers may better understand which strains are most dangerous and discover key determinants in viral pathogenicity. Furthermore, this high-throughput microarray technology can be used to detect a broad spectrum of viruses in one test within a DNA chip.[25]

In addition to nucleic acid-based detection, protein-based technologies, such as protein microarray or protein chip, are other potentially valuable tools for SARS diagnosis. One of the protein chip technologies is based on the surface-enhanced laser desorption/ionization (SELDI) technology.[26,27] The SELDI process is a unique combination and miniaturization of technologies on a single, unified platform. SELDI enables detection and analysis of proteins from complex biological samples, such as sera, directly on protein chip surfaces. This technology is being employed by several groups, including the Health Canada National Microbiology Laboratory, the Beijing Clinical SARS Testing Center and the Genomic Institute of Singapore, in the search for novel protein biomarkers associated with severe acute respiratory syndrome (SARS) (http://www.ciphergen.com).

With the intense efforts by numerous groups around the world, it is expected that numerous new methods for SARS-CoV detection will be forthcoming over the next few months.

ACKNOWLEDGEMENTS

This work is supported by the Hong Kong Research Grants Council Special Grants for SARS Research (CUHK 4508/03M). We would like to thank Prof. Paul Chan for his kind sharing of unpublished data regarding virus culture.

REFERENCES

1. Ksiazek TG, Erdman D, Goldsmith CS, *et al.* A novel coronavirus associated with severe acute respiratory syndrome. *N Engl J Med* 2003;**348**:1953–66.

2. Drosten C, Gunther S, Preiser W, *et al.* Identification of a novel coronavirus in patients with severe acute respiratory syndrome. *N Engl J Med* 2003;**348**:1967–76.

3. Peiris JS, Lai ST, Poon LL, *et al.* Coronavirus as a possible cause of severe acute respiratory syndrome. *Lancet* 2003;**361**:1319–25.

4. Poutanen SM, Low DE, Henry B, *et al.* Identification of severe acute respiratory syndrome in Canada. *N Engl J Med* 2003;**348**:1995–2005.

5. Fouchier RA, Kuiken T, Schutten M, *et al.* Aetiology: Koch's postulates fulfilled for SARS virus. *Nature* 2003;**423**:240.

6. Kuiken T, Fouchier RAM, Schutten M, *et al.* Newly discovered coronavirus as the primary cause of severe acute respiratory syndrome. *Lancet* 2003;**362**:263–70.

7. Peiris JS, Chu CM, Cheng VC, *et al.* Clinical progression and viral load in a community outbreak of coronavirus-associated SARS pneumonia: A prospective study. *Lancet* 2003;**361**:1767–72.

8. Li G, Chen XJ, Xu AL. Profile of specific antibodies to the SARS-associated coronavirus. *N Engl J Med* 2003;**349**:508–9.

9. Tsui SK, Chim SS, Lo YMD, and The Chinese University of Hong Kong Molecular SARS Research Group. Coronavirus genomic-sequence variations and the epidemiology of the severe acute respiratory syndrome. *N Engl J Med* 2003;**349**:187–8.

10. Rota PA, Oberste MS, Monroe SS, *et al.* Characterization of a novel coronavirus associated with severe acute respiratory syndrome. *Science* 2003;**300**:1394–9.

11. Marra MA, Jones SJ, Astell CR, *et al.* The Genome sequence of the SARS-associated coronavirus. *Science* 2003;**300**:1399–404.

12. Poon LL, Wong OK, Luk W, *et al.* Diagnosis of a coronavirus associated with severe acute respiratory syndrome (SARS). *Clin Chem* 2003;**49**:953–5.

13. Ng EKO, Hui DS, Chan KC, *et al.* Quantitative analysis and prognostic implication of SARS-coronavirus RNA in the plasma and serum of patients with severe acute respiratory syndrome. *Clin Chem* 2003;**49**:1976–80.

14. Ng EKO, Ng PC, Hon KLE, *et al.* Serial analysis of the plasma concentration of SARS-coronavirus RNA in pediatric patients with severe acute respiratory syndrome. *Clin Chem* 2003;**49**:2085–8.

15. Kwok S, Higuchi R. Avoiding false positives with PCR. *Nature* 1989;**339**:237–8.

16. Longo MC, Berninger MS, Hartley JL. Use of uracil DNA glycosylase to control carry-over contamination in polymerase chain reactions. *Gene* 1990;**93**:125–8.

17. White PA, Pan Y, Freeman AJ, *et al.* Quantification of hepatitis C virus in human liver and serum samples by using LightCycler reverse transcriptase PCR. *J Clin Microbiol* 2002;**40**:4346–8.

18. Damond F, Descamps D, Farfara I, *et al.* Quantification of proviral load of human immunodeficiency virus type 2 subtypes A and B using real-time PCR. *J Clin Microbiol* 2001;**39**:4264–8.

19. Bustin SA. Absolute quantification of mRNA using real-time reverse transcription polymerase chain reaction assays. *J Mol Endocrinol* 2000;**25**:169–93.

20. Ng EKO, Tsui NB, Lau TK, *et al.* mRNA of placental origin is readily detectable   maternal plasma. *Proc Natl Acad Sci USA* 2003; **100**:4748–53.

21. Chiu, WK, Cheung, PC, Ng, KL, *et al.* Severe acute respiratory syndrome in children: Experience in a regional hospital in Hong Kong. *Pediatr Crit Care Med* 2003;**4**:279–83.

22. Hon KL, Leung CW, Cheng WT, *et al.* Clinical presentations and outcome of severe acute respiratory syndrome in children. *Lancet* 2003;**361**:1701–03.

23. Lee N, Hui D, Wu A, *et al.* A major outbreak of severe acute respiratory syndrome in Hong Kong. *N Engl J Med* 2003;**348**:1986–94.

24. Notomi T, Okayama H, Masubuchi H, *et al.* Loop-mediated isothermal amplification of DNA. *Nucleic Acids Res* 2000;**28**:E63.

25. Wang D, Coscoy L, Zylberberg M, *et al.* Microarray-based detection and genotyping of viral pathogens. *Proc Natl Acad Sci USA* 2002;**99**:15687–92.

26. Issaq HJ, Veenstra TD, Conrads TP, Felschow D. The SELDI-TOF MS approach to proteomics: Protein profiling and biomarker identification. *Biochem Biophys Res Commun* 2002;**292**:587–92.

27. Issaq HJ, Conrads TP, Prieto DA, Tirumalai R, Veenstra TD. SELDI-TOF MS for diagnostic proteomics. *Anal Chem* 2003;**75**:148A–155A.

7

Screening at the Primary Care Setting

Timothy H Rainer

INTRODUCTION

When an outbreak of a novel, highly infectious, potentially lethal illness of unknown etiology, non-specific clinical presentation, unknown clinical course and unknown prognosis first affects both the hospital and community, many challenges face both those who stand at the frontline and those who are responsible for leadership.[1-3] The priorities include staff safety, patient safety, appropriate clinical assessment, disease diagnosis and monitoring, appropriate disposal, constant reassurance and maintaining of morale.

Primary care settings vary considerably both in role, responsibility and organization. They include emergency departments, infectious diseases clinics, public and private outpatient departments and general practitioner facilities. Despite the difference in priority, nevertheless all have a primary role to play to safely, sort patients on a priority basis, and to dispose of patients in the most appropriate fashion.

In this chapter, safety of staff and patients, the early clinical presentation, investigations and decision tree processes for sorting SARS from non-SARS cases will be discussed. The focus is on the experiences and information gained from a newly opened SARS clinic which was resourced and supervised by emergency personnel during an outbreak of SARS. Nevertheless, many principles may be applied to other primary healthcare settings.

Important groups such as children,[4] the elderly,[5] psychiatric cases, pregnant and atypical presentations are all relevant to primary care but will be discussed in other chapters. Therefore, specific issues relating to such groups are not discussed here.

A DYNAMIC SITUATION

When dealing with an outbreak of an unknown, potentially lethal infectious disease which has already affected many colleagues[6] and claimed the lives of frontline staff,[7] staff are frightened[8,9] and the situation updates change by the day. New accurate and inaccurate, relevant and irrelevant information becomes available.[10,11] The three things that staff working in a potentially dangerous environment most desire are calm and objective leadership, personal protection and stability. However, the changes in policy and procedure that inevitably arise challenge both morale and stability. In general, there were several phases in the primary care response to the outbreak. Initially there was little information but within days an area in the emergency department was separated out for assessing and sorting possible SARS cases.[12] Shortly after this, the emergency department was closed for over a week in order to give the hospital a chance to recover from the initial onslaught. Later, the emergency department was opened and the SARS clinic area was moved out of the hospital in order to separate the high risk area from the general emergency department and the rest of the hospital. The aim was to continue processing SARS cases but to try and return the rest of the hospital to normal functioning as soon as possible.

In the crisis, the focus is on SARS and it is easy to forget that patients will still fall ill with all the other common complaints and attend all sorts of primary care facilities for advice and treatment. Decisions regarding the system need to made so that both suspect SARS and other sickness are appropriately treated.

STAFF SAFETY

During the SARS crisis the safest place was not to be in hospital,[13,14] but this was not an option for many staff including those working on the frontline. Staff faced both the physical challenge of contracting the virus and the psychological apprehension. Therefore, measures were needed to minimize the risk of contracting SARS and to meet the psychological needs of staff.

An environment needs to be isolated where patients can be sorted and assessed. There need to be clear, policed entry and exit points with clear protocols for putting on and putting off protective equipment. Figure 1 shows the generally recommended advice given to staff working in the SARS clinic. Figure 2 shows the procedures for putting on and taking off personal protective equipment (PPE), whilst Fig. 3 illustrates the recommended PPE on a staff member. Patients also require advice although there may some modification from the staff recommendation (Fig. 4).

All staff were advised:

- to wash hands with liquid soap before and after patient contact, and after removing of gloves.
- to change gloves between patients and to wash hands.
- to wear a mask in clinic at all times.
- to wear a mask out of hospital if they were in contact with anyone with respiratory symptoms or fever.
- to wear gloves for all direct patient contacts.
- to wear a gown in clinic at all times.
- to wear eye protection gear (e.g. goggles).
- to avoid aerosols and use of nebulizers.
- to clean surfaces regularly with disinfectant.
- to seek medical protection promptly if they have symptoms compatible with SARS (e.g. fever, chills, myalgia, shortness of breath and breathing difficulty).
- to build up good body immunity with proper diet, regular exercise, rest, reduced stress and to avoid smoking.
- to maintain good ventilation.
- to avoid crowded places with poor ventilation.
- to know how to respond when splashed by respiratory secretions (should ask for immediate relief and go washing).
- that, after hand washing, to use paper towel (not elbow) to turn off the tap.
- to know their "Shift Infection Control Officer" who would conduct random audits.

Fig. 1 Health advice offered to staff working in the screening clinic.

When putting on Personal Protective Equipment (PPE)

1. Wash hands
2. Put on cap/face-shield
3. Put on visor/mask
4. Put on gown
5. Put on gloves

Removing PPE (to dispose off dirty gown)

1. Remove cap/face-shield
2. Remove gown
3. Remove glove
4. Wash hands
5. Remove visor/mask
6. Wash hands

Removing PPE (to keep clean gown for re-use)

1. Remove cap/face-shield
2. Remove glove
3. Remove gown — fold inside-out and keep in plastic bag
4. Wash hands
5. Remove visor/mask
6. Wash hands

Fig. 2 Stepwise approach to dressing and removing personal protective equipment (PPE).

Once in the area, there needs to be a clear, linear system through which the patient passes, as they are first offered protective equipment (e.g. face masks); given up to date information (e.g. regarding the illness, common symptoms, process of care and personal hygiene); have their basic observations recorded (e.g. temperature); see a physician for assessment, receive appropriate diagnostic or assessment investigations (e.g. X-rays, blood tests); receive any definitive or non-specific tests; and receive accurate information regarding discharge, referral, follow-up or discharge. It is vital that all doctors and nurses understand the importance of a tidy, linear, orderly method of processing patients. Congestion should be minimized and rooms well ventilated preferably with negative pressure ventilation.

There is little evidence for the optimal level of personal protective equipment that is most appropriate in the early phases of the illness when most patients will seek help. However, advice has been published based on other settings.[15-17] Suggestions range from a minimalist approach,

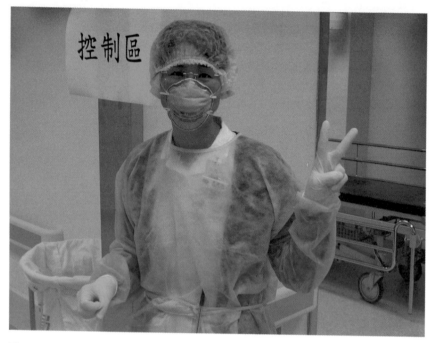

Fig. 3 Staff wearing personal protective equipment.

All patients were advised:

- to wear a mask in clinic at all times.
- to wear a mask out of hospital if they had respiratory symptoms or fever or were in contact with anyone with respiratory symptoms or fever.
- to wash hands with liquid soap before and after patient contact, and after removing gloves.
- to clean surfaces regularly with disinfectant.
- to seek medical protection promptly if they had symptoms compatible with SARS (e.g. fever, chills, myalgia, shortness of breath and breathing difficulty).
- to build up good body immunity with proper diet, regular exercise, rest, reduced stress and to avoid smoking.
- to maintain good ventilation.
- to avoid crowded places with poor ventilation.
- to pay attention to a hygiene information sheet.

Fig. 4 Health advice offered to patients attending the screening clinic.

where staff wear only face masks, wash their hands frequently and take showers if there is any obvious contact; to the maximalist approach where staff wear hats, goggles, shields, N95 or N100 face masks, gowns, gloves, and covering for shoes. The minimalist approach has been criticized as it leaves staff over exposed, whilst the efforts required to remove the equipment in the maximalist approach are also not without risk.

Other practical questions have been raised for which there are no definitive answers. Should staff use stethoscopes to examine all patients and should the stethoscope be cleansed between each patient? If so, what level of cleansing is required? Should the blood pressure cuff be covered with a disposable plastic bag, and should this be changed for each patient or only for those patients with pyrexia? How far should patients lying on trolleys or seated on chairs be spaced next to one another?

The best current evidence is that most patients have low infectivity in the first week of symptoms and that therefore staff are at relatively low risk during this phase.[18] However, primary care does not limit the time when patients can seek help and primary care physicians will screen patients no matter how long the time from onset of symptoms. Therefore vigilance is required at all times.

In Hong Kong, after the SARS clinic was opened and protocols put in place, only three primary care staff members contracted SARS, one from a family member and not from work, one after admission to hospital, and only one most likely contracted the illness at work. Therefore the following protocol is probably quite safe. In our experience of screening over 1000 cases, we had over 100 confirmed cases of SARS. We found that there were no known cases of secondary spread amongst the suspicious cases followed at home with strict quarantine instructions, although this requires further detailed investigation.

STAFF MORALE AND LEADERSHIP

During the outbreak, it was important that staff worked as a team. The team needed frequent, clear, calm information, sensible decisions and protocols, flexibility and constant encouragement. Staff needed to see leaders working at the frontline, sharing the risk, setting an example, staying calm, and maintaining morale. Staff needed to know the truth but needed information in quantities that could be digested.

SARS SCREENING CLINIC

An outbreak in the Prince of Wales hospital was evident as early as 8 March 2003, and in response to this crisis, a SARS clinic based in the emergency department of the Prince of Wales Hospital was opened on

12 March 2003.[12] Infectious disease surveillance with daily follow-up is not the primary role of an emergency department. Nevertheless, in times of crisis, it is appropriate that specialties are flexible, and modify the scope of their responsibilities to support the system as a whole. In this crisis, it was appropriate that the emergency department take on this role, especially as the overall attendance rate plummeted, and few emergency staff went ill. Other primary care settings may be similarly challenged.

CASE DEFINITION OF SARS AND PRESENTATION IN THE PRIMARY CARE SETTING

According to WHO, SARS is *suspected* in a person with a high fever (>38°C), AND one or more respiratory symptoms (e.g. cough, shortness of breath or difficulty in breathing), AND close contact with a person previously diagnosed with SARS.[19,20] A *probable* case of SARS is when an individual meets the criteria of a suspected case but then develops pneumonic change on chest X-ray. At present, it is virtually impossible to confirm SARS at the primary care setting, although one can make a good guess!

The current WHO case definition for suspect SARS has a sensitivity of 25%.[12] The reason for the poor sensitivity is because ALL criteria have to be fulfilled to meet the case definition. In the first week of illness, when surveillance should be high and the net cast wide enough to catch nearly all "suspect" cases for close monitoring and follow-up, many patients have a contact history, systemic symptoms, respiratory or abdominal symptoms, but do not have a recordable temperature >38°C, cough, shortness of breath or difficulty in breathing. Therefore by definition they are not suspect. If the criteria were followed closely, then many patients would not be suspected of SARS and could possibly be discharged without surveillance. All the criteria for suspect SARS are carried forward to the case definition for probable SARS. Therefore, the weakness in the definition also carries forward. Many patients in the primary care setting have systemic or gastrointestinal symptoms, a contact history and pneumonic change on X-ray, yet have no temperature recording >38°C, and no respiratory symptoms of cough, shortness of breath or difficulty in breathing. Therefore by definition they are not probable cases, yet common sense dictates that they probably have SARS and should be isolated as "probable" cases. Thus, the WHO case definitions as they currently stand are probably not practically useful for early screening of SARS.

After an incubation period of 2 to 16 days,[13] patients with SARS present initially with non-specific systemic, respiratory or gastrointestinal symptoms (Table 1).[12] Fever, chills, malaise and myalgia are amongst the commonest symptoms and were also most discriminatory during the outbreak. Although cough is common in SARS cases, it was actually more common in non-SARS (72%) than SARS cases, and therefore was not a useful discriminatory symptom. Shortness of breath, whilst more common in SARS than non-SARS cases, only affected 12% cases. Therefore, respiratory symptoms are of limited usefulness in the early assessment. Vomiting, diarrhea and abdominal pain occurred in a limited number of SARS cases. Although many SARS cases present with pneumonia, no more than 1% complained of pleuritic chest pain.

On examination, very few of these patients have any clinical signs in the early phase and therefore, the diagnosis in the primary care setting based on clinical criteria alone is almost impossible! Basal crackles have been noted in patients after admission to hospital,[13] but despite thorough assessment in the primary care setting, there was little evidence of this in SARS patients with pneumonia.[12] Sore throat, lymphadenopathy and skin rashes are also absent. Therefore the early presentation of SARS is

Table 1 Clinical Symptoms in the First Few Days of Illness[7]

Fever	81%*
Cough	64%
Chills	54%*
Sore throat	35%
Malaise	34%*
Myalgia	27%*
Sputum	26%
Rhinorrhea	26%
Headache	26%
Rigor	12%*
Shortness of breath	12%*
Diarrhea	7%*
Vomiting	6%*
Dizziness	6%
Abdominal pain	4%
Loss of appetite	5%*
Chest pain	1%

* Significantly more common than non-SARS cases.

very non-specific and it is difficult to discriminate other common viral causes from SARS. It is only the outbreak and the high probability of SARS which helps primary care physicians make the diagnosis at all!

Two distinctly different contexts exist — during an outbreak and outwith an outbreak. During an outbreak, the likelihood of SARS infection is high, and so SARS should be suspected in any patient who presents with non-specific systemic, respiratory or gastrointestinal symptoms. Patients with non-infectious illness are reluctant to attend hospital and so numbers of attendances decrease. This frees frontline staff to open and man a new clinic such as a SARS clinic.

Once the outbreak has ended, the detection of SARS is much more difficult. The early presentation of SARS is vague and non-specific. Is the illness dormant in the community waiting to emerge at any time or is it in fact not present at all? Differentiating SARS from other non-SARS causes of non-specific systemic, respiratory and gastrointestinal symptoms is virtually impossible when SARS is not present in the community. It is neither practical nor feasible to follow up on a daily basis and arrange daily X-rays for every patient with fever, et cetera. In reality we have to be vigilant but assume that SARS is not present.

TIPS FOR PRIMARY CARE DOCTORS TO DIAGNOSE SARS

At the primary care setting, it is often difficult, if not impossible, to diagnose SARS on the spot during the first encounter. The trick of the trade is to continue observation for a few days consecutively. All patients should have a pulse rate, systolic and diastolic blood pressure, respiratory rate, temperature recording and oxygen saturation at every presentation at clinic. Although patients with SARS have a more pronounced tachycardia and higher temperature reading than those patients without SARS, nevertheless less than 50% of SARS cases with radiological evidence of pneumonia have a temperature >38°C both at first attendance and during subsequent clinic follow-up prior to admission.[12] Although lower respiratory symptoms are a main feature of the WHO case definition for SARS,[8,9] SARS patients with pneumonia do not have a raised respiratory rate in the early phase of the illness.[12]

Complete blood and differential counts, urea and electrolytes, liver function tests, urea and coagulation profile may be requested early in the course of the illness.[28,29] Although lymphopenia is a cardinal feature of

SARS patients, later in the illness and after admission to hospital, its value in the early phase is not clear. About 50% of symptomatic cases with lymphopenia attending our clinic subsequently developed SARS. The other 50% made a full recovery with resolution of the lymphopenia after 48 hours or so, and demonstrated no positive serological evidence of SARS. Some patients had profound lymphopenia (0.2×10^9/L), yet recovered within 48 hours. Therefore lymphopenia should be a reason for isolation and regular follow-up but not for admission to a SARS triage or cohort ward.

In the context of an outbreak, a contact history, clinical criteria and elevated temperature readings alone yield a sensitivity of detecting SARS in the primary care setting of only 80%. However, the addition of daily chest X-ray[30–32] or high resolution computerized tomography,[33–35] improves decision making to give a sensitivity of 100% and a positive predictive value of 60%. Chest X-rays requested in the first 100 SARS cases presenting to a SARS clinic showed a variety of presentations, including unifocal (Fig. 5), multifocal (Fig. 6) and diffuse (Fig. 7)

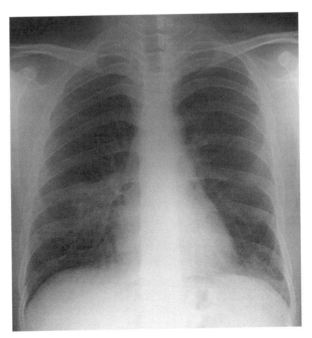

Fig. 5 Frontal chest radiograph showing an area of air space opacification in the right lower zone in a patient with SARS. (*Courtesy of Department of Diagnostic Radiology and Organ Imaging, CUHK*).

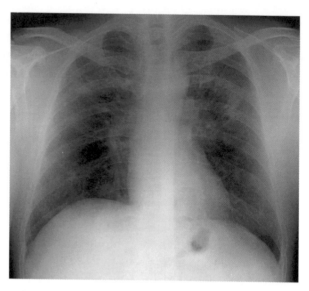

Fig. 6 Frontal chest radiograph showing multiple areas of consolidation in both lung fields in a patient with SARS. (*Courtesy of Department of Diagnostic Radiology and Organ Imaging, CUHK*).

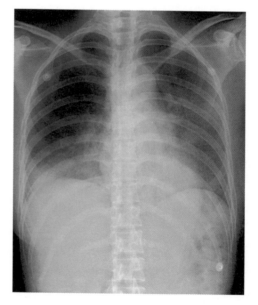

Fig. 7 Frontal chest radiograph showing diffuse areas of consolidation in both lower and left mid zones in a patient with SARS. (*Courtesy of Department of Diagnostic Radiology and Organ Imaging, CUHK*).

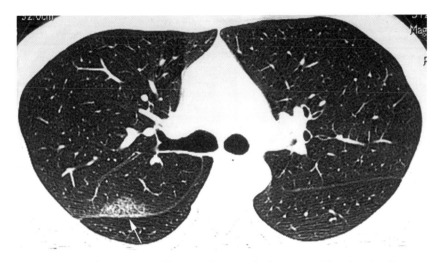

Fig. 8 HRCT shows a small area of ground-glass opacification in the posterior segment of the right upper lobe in a patient with SARS (arrow). (*Courtesy of Department of Diagnostic Radiology and Organ Imaging, CUHK*).

pneumonia.[9,12] High resolution computerized tomography (HRCT) was requested in some patients with persistent symptoms and elevated temperature recordings but normal chest radiographs. In SARS cases, HRCT showed a typical area of ground-glass opacification (Fig. 8). Some patients with normal radiographs (Fig. 9a) have retrocardiac (Fig. 9b) or retro-diaphragmatic (Fig. 9c) lesions evident on HRCT.

LABORATORY DIAGNOSIS OF SARS

Now that the virus has been isolated, diagnostic tests of variable sensitivity and specificity begin to emerge. Nevertheless, there are no accurate tests that were useful for decision making in the primary care setting during the SARS crisis of March to May 2003. This situation is likely to change in the near future as rapid tests become available that have high sensitivity and specificity early in the course of the illness. The virus can be isolated from the sputum, nasopharyngeal aspirates, throat wash, urine and from lung biopsy, and after incubation may be identified by electron microscopy.[18,22,24] Antibodies to SARS-CoV may be detected in serum using immunofluorescence assay (IFA) and subsequently detected by enzyme-linked immunosorbent assay (ELISA). However, results from

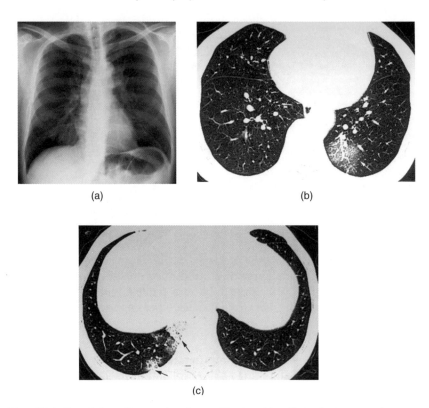

(a)   (b)

(c)

Fig. 9(a) Frontal radiograph of a patient with clinical signs and symptoms highly suggestive of SARS but no obvious radiological abnormality. (*Courtesy of Department of Diagnostic Radiology and Organ Imaging, CUHK*). **(b)** HRCT in the same patient taken several hours after the radiograph shows ground-glass opacification in the posterior basal segment of the left lower lobe (arrow). The abnormality is situated behind the heart which makes it difficult to identify it on a frontal CXR. (*Courtesy of Department of Diagnostic Radiology and Organ Imaging, CUHK*). **(c)** HRCT in another SARS patient with a normal frontal chest radiograph shows consolidations in the basal segments of the right lower lobe (arrows). Note its retrodiaghragmatic location which makes it difficult to identify it on a frontal CXR. (*Courtesy of Department of Diagnostic Radiology and Organ Imaging, CUHK*).

these tests are not useful for the emergency department or primary care clinics as their positivity is delayed. Reverse transcriptase polymerase chain reaction (RT–PCR) on respiratory, urine, stool and blood samples may offer rapid, accurate diagnostic tests in the near future.[36, 37] (see chapter on Laboratory Diagnosis).

DECISION TREES AND DISPOSAL POLICIES

In theory every suspected case of SARS should be isolated. However, where should undiagnosed but suspect SARS cases be isolated and for how long? Should all suspect cases be admitted to hospital, a practice clearly entertained in some countries? If so, some suspected cases will have the illness and many would not. To admit or cohort all suspect cases into a communal area will be to subject non-SARS patients to contact SARS patients resulting in non-SARS cases eventually contracting the illness. This clearly challenges the first principle of safety first. Many patients who developed SARS probably did so after admission to hospital. Whilst there is no good data to confirm this, nevertheless this remains highly likely. Hospitals are dangerous places!

The alternative is to delay or not admit suspect cases to hospital at all. Many of the patients attending our emergency SARS clinic were hospital colleagues and friends who presented with non-specific symptoms. The last thing anyone wanted to do was admit friends and colleagues who may contract the illness after admission. However, to discharge these cases into the community was to risk spreading the illness further in the community. SARS was also a dangerously progressive illness for which monitoring was essential to identify those who might need intensive care or alternative strategies, such as high dose therapy or ribavirin. Returning patients to the community also involved risk. Therefore, there were no easy answers to any of these questions but one key principle is individual isolation and another is close monitoring.

There are a number of other reasons favoring a delay in hospital admission. Firstly, there is no evidence of any patient with normal physiology (pulse rate, blood pressure respiratory rate and oxygen saturation) deteriorating to require intensive care or dying within 24 hours. All take days to deteriorate significantly. Secondly, although there may be political pressure for the public to come forward early in order to receive curative treatment, there is no good evidence to show that such treatment exists. Although some patients clearly deteriorate, benefit from intensive care and may benefit from limited courses of steroids or other definitive treatment, yet many patients have recovered fully without steroids, antiviral therapy or any other definitive therapy.

Therefore, it is not urgent that all suspect cases are admitted to infectious triage wards or even that many of these cases should be admitted at all. However, all suspect cases should be followed up and monitored regularly (every 24 to 48 hours) at a "SARS" clinic or specified area. All cases should receive advice regarding personal isolation, personal protection and personal hygiene (see Fig. 4).

Every individual situation should be considered in its own right. It may not be wise for a suspect case to return home to stay with other family members especially with elderly or chronically ill residents. Some cases may not be sensible or alert to their own condition.

Should the patient be given the choice? Many of us live in a free world where patient rights and preferences are regarded very highly. However, the risk to the community and society also has major economic and other implications if suspect cases wander everywhere. In practice the vast majority of patients are wise and sensible, appreciate the risks, evaluate seriously their own personal circumstances and make sensible judgments based on the relative risk to themselves, their family and community. Many chose to isolate themselves alone at home, in another flat, in a hotel room, in an office or elsewhere until their status was more clearly defined.

Two broad opinions have therefore emerged — those who favour home isolation and those who favor hospital isolation. Neither will be correct in every case, but each has its merits and each case should be considered in its own rights.

Guidelines for screening high-risk contact and low risk non-contact subjects have recently been published.[10,11,19,20] We offered modified guidelines based on our local experience (Fig. 10; Ref. 12). All of our subjects were likely to have some contact with a SARS case and so, unlike the general population where there may be no known contact, our cohort were at high risk of contracting the disease. In view of the fact that symptoms were often vague, that high temperature readings may be less common in the early development, that clinical examination of the mouth, throat and chest usually revealed no abnormality even in patients with advanced stages of SARS-pneumonia, the importance of regular chest X-rays with or without CT cannot be over-emphasized.

Hospital Admission Criteria

The initial primary criteria for admission to a hospital clearing ward was EITHER a history of close contact with a SARS patient in the previous

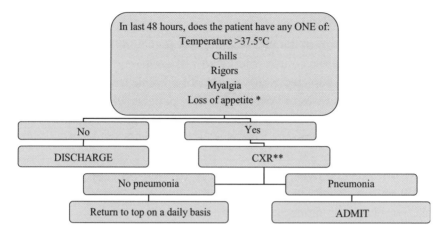

In last 48 hours, does the patient have any ONE of:
Temperature >37.5°C
Chills
Rigors
Myalgia
Loss of appetite *

No → DISCHARGE

Yes → CXR**

No pneumonia → Return to top on a daily basis

Pneumonia → ADMIT

* Note that in this cohort, systemic symptoms alone are sufficient to produce a model that is highly sensitive and specific. However, as other studies have emphasized respiratory (cough and shortness of breath) and gastrointestinal symptoms (vomiting, abdominal pain), these should not be discounted.

** Consider high resolution computerized tomography for cases with ≥ 3 days persistent symptoms but normal chest radiograph.

Fig. 10 Guidelines on predicting SARS-pneumonia.

10 days, fever and chills/rigors, and documented pyrexia >38°C, OR a history of fever, chills and rigors and any one of four abnormalities: an oxygen saturation of <95%; abnormal chest radiograph; unstable hemodynamics; or abnormal blood results.

It quickly became evident that many patients attending the clinic had brief transient episodes of lymphopenia or thrombocytopenia which resolved in 24 to 48 hours. Whether these patients had minor presentations of SARS was not clear at the time, but subsequent follow-up has shown that less than 5% have SARS-CoV positive serology. These patients did not develop SARS pneumonia and appeared to have a typical viral episode that quickly resolved. Therefore, the majority probably did not have SARS but rather another of the non-specific, common viral causes of upper respiratory tract infections. These cases of suspect SARS were not admitted to hospital, but were advised to isolate themselves from their families. Many staff moved into hospital accommodation or hotels. Only probable cases of SARS were admitted to a hospital ward.

Follow-up Criteria

As little was known of the illness in the first two months of the outbreak in Hong Kong, and as our medical staff were severely depleted because colleagues had contracted SARS, it was not possible let alone prudent to admit all suspect cases to hospital. The few patients who were admitted to hospital were rapidly discharged the next day, only to return to our clinic for further follow-up. Therefore, patients were followed up daily after first attendance if there was a contact history, one or more symptoms, documented pyrexia >37.5°C on at least one occasion, a normal or indeterminate chest radiograph, or abnormal investigations (e.g. leucopenia, lymphopenia, monocytosis or thrombocytosis). Patients were given hygiene advice and a follow-up appointment for the next day.

Discharge Criteria

Patients were discharged after first attendance if they had vague or no symptoms, no pyrexia, a normal radiograph and normal laboratory investigations. They were given hygiene advice and advised to return if they experienced systemic, respiratory or gastrointestinal symptoms and a fever. Symptomatic patients were followed up daily and discharged only after 48 hours of remaining asymptomatic, with no documented pyrexia and normal chest radiographs and laboratory tests.

CONCLUSION

The lessons in this chapter are really learnt from the context of an outbreak. With the global spread of disease, it is likely that other outbreaks will occur and that healthcare settings will be faced with the similar dilemma of screening symptomatic staff, patients and members of the community who have had close contact with SARS-pneumonia patients after a SARS outbreak.

This chapter describes the clinical features and process of care in a screening clinic which provided a safe environment for staff, patients and their contacts with no secondary infections. Hospitals are dangerous places for patients who do not have SARS. Unless facilities for mass isolation rooms are available, it may be better to quarantine patients at home, in camps or in empty government properties in order to avoid passing on the illness to SARS-free cases. The early phase of the illness is characterized by a non-specific systemic (such as fever, myalgia and chills), gastrointestinal and respiratory symptoms. Documented fever is often not possible despite the presence of pneumonic change on X-ray.

One of the greatest challenges will be to make an early, accurate diagnosis of SARS. Once this is done, patients may be quarantined with other SARS cases without danger of cross infection. Therefore, both the discovery and confirmed value of a rapid, early, accurate, bedside test is essential for early diagnosis and appropriate management.

ACKNOWLEDGEMENTS

Much gratitude goes to frontline hospital staff who put their lives on the line to serve patients and colleagues during this outbreak, and who helped to collect quality information that will guide clinicians' decision making in the future.

REFERENCES

1. Cameron PA, Rainer TH, Smit P DeV. The SARS epidemic: Lessons for Australia. *Med J Aus* 2003;**178**(10):478–479.

2. Cameron PA, Rainer TH. Update on Emerging Infections: News from the Centers for Disease Control and Prevention. *Annals of Emergency Medicine* 2003;**42**:1–8.

3. Cameron PA. The Plague within: An Australian doctor's experience of SARS in Hong Kong. *Med J Aus* 2003;**178**(10):512–513.

4. Hon KLE, Leung CW, Cheng WTF, *et al.* Research letters: Clinical presentations and outcome of severe acute respiratory syndrome in children. *Lancet* 2003;**361**:1701–3.

5. Action Group for Elders and SARS 2003 http://ageing.hku.hk.

6. Wong RSM. Severe acute respiratory syndrome in a doctor working at the Prince of Wales Hospital. *Hong Kong Med J* 2003;**9**:202–5.

7. Reilley B, Van Herp M, Sermand D, Dentico N. SARS and Carlo Urbani. *N Engl J Med* 2003;**348**:1951–2.

8. Masur H, Emanuel E, Lane HC. Severe acute respiratory syndrome: Providing care in the face of uncertainty. *JAMA* 2003;**289**:10–12.

9. Razum O, Becher H, Kapaun A and Junghanss T. SARS, lay epidemiology and fear. *Lancet* 2003 http://image.thelancet.com/extras/03cor4133web.pdf.

10. CDC. Updated interim US case definition for severe acute respiratory syndrome (SARS). 2003. (Accessed at http://www.cdc.gov/ncidod/sars on May 23).

11. Ho W, the Hong Kong Hospital Authority Working Group on SARS and the Central Committee on Infection Control. Guidelines on management of severe acute respiratory syndrome (SARS). *Lancet* 2003;**361**:1313.

12. Rainer TH, Cameron PA, Smit DeV, *et al.* Evaluation of the WHO criteria for identifying patients with severe acute respiratory syndrome (SARS) Pneumonia out of hospital: Prospective observational study. *BMJ* 2003;**326**:1354–8.

13. Lee N, Hui D, Wu A, *et al.* A major outbreak of severe acute respiratory syndrome (SARS) in Hong Kong. *N Eng J Med* 2003;**348**:1986–94.

14. Booth CM, Matukas LM, Tomlinson GA, *et al.* Clinical features and short-term outcomes of 144 patients with SARS in the Greater Toronto area. *JAMA-Express* 2003;**289**(21)1–9.

15. Li TST, Buckley TA, Yap FHY, Sung JJY, Joynt GM. Severe acute respiratory syndrome (SARS): Infection control. *Lancet* 2003;**361**:1386.

16. Seto WH, Tsang D, Yung RWH, *et al.* Effectiveness of precautions against droplets and contact in prevention of nosocomial transmission of severe acute respiratory syndrome (SARS). *Lancet* 2003;**361**:1519–20.

17. Yang W. Severe acute respiratory syndrome (SARS): Infection control. *Lancet* 2003;**361**:1386–7.

18. Peiris JSM, Lai ST, Poon LLM, *et al.* Coronavirus as a possible cause of severe acute respiratory syndrome. *Lancet* 2003;**361**:1319–25.

19. WHO. Severe acute respiratory syndrome. *Wkly Epidemiol Rec* No. 14. 2003;**78**:97–120.

20. WHO. Case definitions for surveillance of severe acute respiratory syndrome (SARS). (Accessed at http://www.who.int/csr/sars/casedefinition/en/).

21. Brown EG and Tetro JA. Comparative analysis of the SARS coronavirus genome: A good start to a long journey. *Lancet* 2003 http://image.thelancet.com/extras/03cmt124web.pdf.

22. Drosten C, Gunther S, Preiser W, *et al.* Identification of a novel coronavirus in patients with severe acute respiratory syndrome. *N Eng J Med* 2003;**348**:1967–76.

23. Falsey AR, Walsh EE. Novel coronavirus and severe acute respiratory syndrome. *Lancet* 2003 (accessed at http://image.thelancet.com/extras/03cmt87web.pdf).

24. Ksiazek TG, Erdman D, Goldsmith C, *et al.* A novel coronavirus associated with severe acute respiratory syndrome. *N Eng J Med* 2003; **348**:1953–66.

25. Rota PA, Oberste MS, Monroe SS, *et al.* Characterization of a novel coronavirus associated with severe acute respiratory syndrome. *Sciencexpress.* 2003 www.sciencexpress.org/1May2003/Page1/10.1126/science.1085952.

26. Ruan Y-J, Wei CL, Ee LA, *et al.* Comparative full-length genome sequence analysis of 14 SARS coronavirus isolates and common mutations associated with putative origins of infection. *Lancet* 2003 http://image.thelancet.com/extras/03art4454web.pdf.

27. Marra MA, Jones SJM, Astell CR, *et al.* The genome sequence of the SARS-associated coronavirus. *Sciencexpress.* 2003 www.sciencexpress.org/1May2003/Page1/10.1126/science.1085953.

28. Yuen E, Kam CW, Rainer TH. Role of absolute lymphocyte count in the screening of patients with suspected SARS. *Emerg Med* 2003 (In press).

29. Wong RSM, Wu A, To KF, *et al.* Haematological manifestations of patients with severe acute respiratory syndrome: Retrospective analysis. *BMJ* 2003 (In press).

30. Wong KT, Antonio GE, Hui DSC, Lee N, Yuen EH, Wu A, Leung CB, Rainer TH, *et al.* Radiological appearances of severe acute respiratory syndrome. *J Hong Kong Coll Radiol* 2003;**6**:4–6.

31. Wong KT, Antonio GE, Hui DSC, Lee N, Yuen EHY, Wu A, Leung CB, Rainer TH, *et al.* Radiographic appearances and pattern of progression of severe acute respiratory syndrome (SARS): A study of 138 patients. *Radiology* 2003:**228**(2); 401–406 [Epub ahead of print].

32. Antonio GE, Wong KT, Hui DSC Lee N, Yuen EHY, Wu A, Leung CB, Rainer TH, *et al.* Pictorial Essay: Imaging of severe acute respiratory syndrome in Hong Kong. *Am J Roentgenol* (in press). Preview on-line at http://www.arrs.org.

33. Antonio GE, Wong KT, Hui DSC, Wu A, Lee N, Yuen EHY, Leung CB, Rainer TH, *et al.* Thin-section computed tomography in severe acute respiratory syndrome (SARS) patients following hospital discharge: Preliminary experience. *Radiology* 2003; June 12 [Epub ahead of print].

34. Wong KT, Antonio GE, Hui DSC, Lee N, Yuen EHY, Wu A, Leung CB, Rainer TH, *et al.* Thin-section CT of severe acute respiratory syndrome: Evaluation of 73 patients exposed to or with the disease. *Radiology* 2003: **228**(2); 395–400 [Epub ahead of print].

35. Antonio GE, Wong KT, Hui DSC, Wu A, Lee N, Yuen EHY, Leung CB, Rainer TH, *et al.* Early progress thin-section computed tomography in severe acute respiratory syndrome: Initial experience. *Radiology* 2003 (In press).

36. Poon LL, Wong OK, Luk W, *et al.* Rapid diagnosis of a coronavirus associated with severe acute respiratory syndrome (SARS). *Clin Chem* 2003;**49**:953–5.

37. Ng EKO, Hui DS, Chan KC, *et al.* Quantitative analysis and prognostic implication of SARS-coronavirus RNA in the plasma and serum of patients with severe acute respiratory syndrome. *Clin Chem* 2003; (In press).

8

Imaging in Severe Acute Respiratory Syndrome

KT Wong, Gregory E Antonio, Anil T Ahuja

INTRODUCTION

The role of radiology in the diagnosis and management of Severe Acute Respiratory Syndrome (SARS) is well established. Imaging is a major diagnostic component of both WHO and CDC guidelines.[1,2] During the initial outbreak there was no laboratory test to quickly establish the diagnosis of SARS and the diagnosis was made using clinical, imaging and hematological criteria. At the time of writing this chapter, virological tests are becoming available although their sensitivity and specificity have yet to be definitively established in a prospective study.

During the three-month epidemic, over 340 cases of SARS were treated at the Prince of Wales Hospital, Hong Kong and imaging played an important role in the diagnosis, management and follow-up after discharge of SARS patients. This chapter is aimed at sharing, the authors experience on the role and relevant findings of imaging in SARS.

ROLE OF IMAGING MODALITIES

As in other chest infections, chest radiography and thin slice or high-resolution computed tomography (HRCT) of the thorax are the two major imaging investigations used in SARS.

Chest Radiograph

The primary objective of the presentation chest radiograph is to assist in diagnosis by demonstrating lung parenchymal changes suggesting infection and by excluding important diagnostic negatives such as pneumothorax, empyema, mass lesions or lymphadenopathy. This can then be compared with progress radiographs to assess disease progression and responses to treatment.[3] A lack of disease response as seen on the chest radiograph is an indicator of treatment failure, which may necessitate more vigorous therapy, addition of new drugs or ventilatory support/intensive care (ICU) admission. The frontal chest radiograph, the posteroanterior view, is the initial imaging investigation for suspected cases of SARS. Lateral projection radiographs do not contribute to additional information in this situation.

High Resolution Computed Tomography

High resolution CT, with its superior resolution for lung abnormalities, is an important accessory imaging tool for the diagnosis of SARS. High resolution CT (1 mm slice thickness) can be used instead of the conventional contrast-enhanced CT (7 to 10 mm thickness), since lymphadenopathy and pleural effusions are not present in SARS.[4] HRCT is indicated in patients with high clinical suspicion but a normal initial chest radiograph.[4] HRCT can also be used to monitor disease progress in patients who have failed to respond to treatment , as well as ICU patients.

The imaging algorithm for the use of HRCT for suspected cases of SARS is presented in Fig. 1. Patients with clinical suspicion of SARS are initially investigated with a frontal chest radiograph. If there is a definite abnormality on the presentation chest radiograph, especially if the abnormality is new when compared with previous radiographs, further imaging will not required for diagnosis and treatment may be started. If the presentation chest radiograph is normal but the clinical features strongly suggest SARS, HRCT of the thorax is used to detect a possible occult disease.

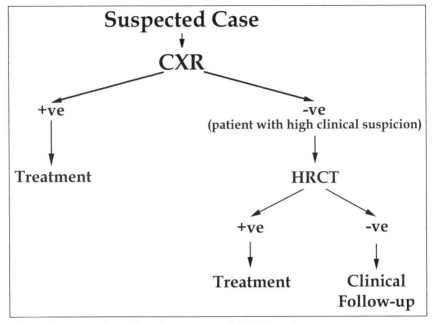

Fig. 1 Imaging algorithm for suspected SARS patients.

Lesions that can be missed on the presentation chest radiographs are those:

- hidden behind dense breast shadows;
- anterior or posterior to the heart;
- behind the hemi-diaphragm.

In an epidemic situation, an abnormality seen only with HRCT coupled with a strong clinical history is adequate for the diagnosis of SARS. However at the end of the epidemic, sporadic cases occur mainly in the elderly. These patients have less clear-cut symptoms and/or contact history, and probable underlying pulmonary disease. The chest radiographs are difficult to interpret and the demand on HRCT may increase. However, because of the non-specific nature of the HRCT findings of SARS, interpretation of HRCT detected abnormalities remains difficult in some cases.

IMAGING FEATURES

The radiographic features for SARS are non-specific. The radiographic changes reflect the pulmonary pathology and its progression. These follow along the same line as most pneumonitis i.e. there is an initial focal area of interstitial inflammation, followed by outpouring of exudate resulting in consolidation, at the same time spreading to other areas and/or becoming confluent. Finally, in most cases resolution begins which may leave behind a fibrotic scar.

There are several radiographic signs that are consistently present in SARS at initial diagnosis. These include[3] (Figs. 2 and 3):

- the majority (78%) of patients have air-space opacification of variable extent;
- lower zone (65%) and peripheral lung fields (75%) are more commonly involved;
- unifocal involvement (54.6%) is more common than multi-focal/bilateral disease;
- cavitation, lymphadenopathy and pleural effusion are absent.

The initial CXR are normal in 22% of patients.[3] If these patients have clinical signs and symptoms highly suggestive of SARS, HRCT should be

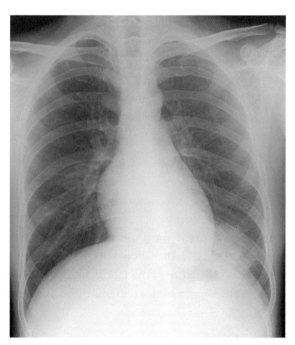

Fig. 2 Frontal chest radiograph of a 28-year-old SARS patient shows ill-defined focal consolidation in left lower zone at presentation.

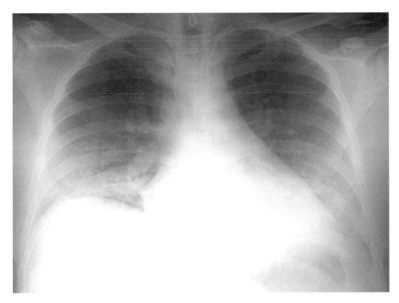

Fig. 3 Frontal chest radiograph of a 32-year-old SARS patient shows multi-focal bilateral air-space opacification in both lower zones at clinical presentation.

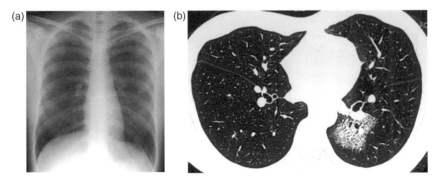

Fig. 4 (a) Frontal chest radiograph at presentation in a 30-year-old female with SARS which is normal. (b) HRCT reveals area of ground-glass opacification in apical segment of left lower lobe. The paraspinal location is a common blind-spot on conventional chest radiograph.

performed which may detect early lung parenchymal changes (Fig. 4). Subsequent follow-up radiographs in this group of patients all show air-space opacification in a couple of days. From then on, radiographs are used as one of the parameters to monitor disease progression and assess the appropriateness of treatment.

During the epidemic, the majority of patients with SARS have abnormal chest radiograph on presentation, and further imaging, such as HRCT, is not necessary for the diagnosis. HRCT of the thorax is reserved for patients with a high clinical index of suspicion of SARS but a negative presentation chest radiograph. The importance of strong clinical correlation must be emphasized since the HRCT findings themselves are non-specific. High resolution computed tomography will probably show non-specific lung changes that are indistinguishable from SARS if used on patients with other forms of lower respiratory tract infection. Interestingly, during the epidemic, for patients with minor symptoms, such as an upper respiratory tract infection, and a generally low index of clinical suspicion, HRCT was invariably negative.[4] These involved mostly healthcare workers in the hospital, who were in a high state of anxiety.

Although non-specific, there are HRCT findings that are consistently present in SARS patients. These common imaging features on HRCT include[4,5] (Figs. 5 and 6):

- ground-glass opacification with or without consolidation;
- lower lobe predilection;
- peripheral/subpleural location of lesions;

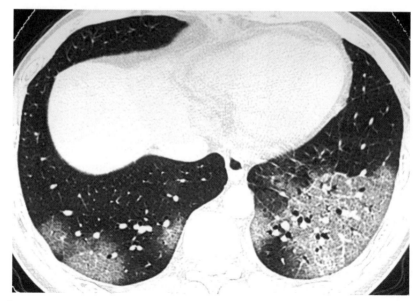

Fig. 5 HRCT of a 29-year-old SARS patient shows multiple peripheral/subpleural ground-glass opacification in both lower lobes.

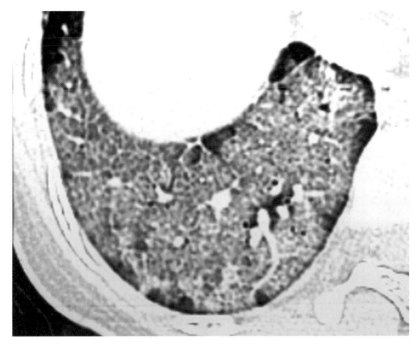

Fig. 6 HRCT of a 32-year-old SARS patient shows ground-glass opacification with thickened interlobular septa and intralobular interstitium (crazy-paving appearances).

- thickening of the intralobular interstitium or interlobular septa within areas of ground-glass opacification. In florid cases, a "crazy-paving" pattern may be seen;
- absence of cavitation, calcification, lymphadenopathy or pleural effusion.

The chest radiographic and HRCT appearances of SARS are indistinguishable from other causes of atypical pneumonia such as mycoplasma, chlamydia and legionella.[6-10] There is also much overlap in radiological features with other types of viral pneumonia in adults.[11] Since imaging alone cannot differentiate SARS from other atypical pneumonias, clinical and laboratory information is indispensable for diagnosis of SARS.[12]

PROGRESS MONITORING AND TREATMENT RESPONSE

In some institutions, patients with a confirmed diagnosis of SARS may be treated initially with a combination of ribavirin and corticosteroid.[12] For patients not responsive to the first line treatment, other forms of therapy such as pulse intravenous methylprednisolone and convalescent serum may be used. Serial chest radiographs play an important role in patient management during the treatment period, as radiographic deterioration is one of the parameters for more aggressive treatment.

During treatment, four different patterns of radiographic progression are observed[3]:

Type 1 — radiographic deterioration to a peak followed by improvement, which is the most commonly encountered pattern (70.5%) (Fig. 7);

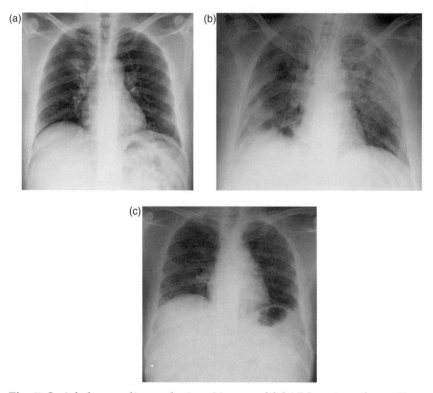

Fig. 7 Serial chest radiographs in a 31-year-old SARS patient shows Type 1 progression pattern during treatment. (a) Frontal CXR at presentation shows focal consolidation in right upper zone. (b) Frontal CXR 10 days later shows confluent bilateral air-space opacification (patient is intubated). (c) Subsequent CXR another 12 days later shows marked improvement in extent of consolidation (patient is successfully weaned off ventilator).

Type 2 — fluctuating radiographic response with at least two peaks during the treatment period (17.5%);
Type 3 — static radiographic appearances with no obvious peak deterioration (7%); and
Type 4 — progressive radiographic deterioration (5%).

In general, patients with Type 4 progression pattern have the worst prognosis in terms of mortality and intensive care admission rate.

Serial chest radiographs are particularly important in the intensive care setting to detect complications of barotrauma such as pneumothorax and pneumo-mediastinum (Figs. 8 and 9). This is in addition to the spontaneous pneumothorax that occurs in SARS patients prior to ventilation. 12% of SARS patients develop spontaneous pneumomediastinum and 20% have evidence of ARDS (Fig. 10) over a period of 3 weeks.[13]

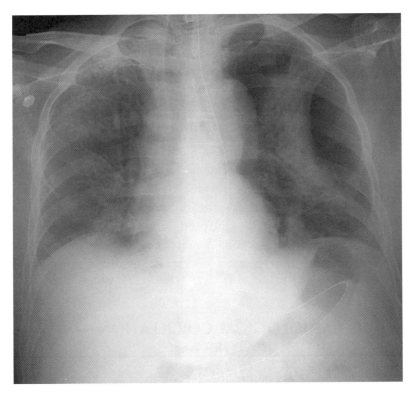

Fig. 8 Frontal chest radiograph in a 54-year-old SARS patient developed spontaneous left pneumothorax which required subsequent thoracocentesis.

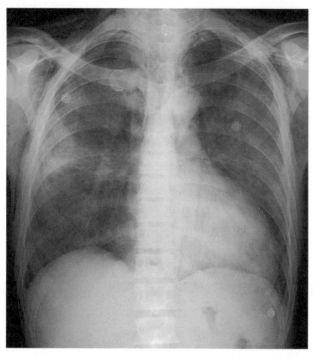

Fig. 9 Frontal chest radiograph in a 33-year-old SARS patient shows the presence of pneumomediastinum and surgical emphysema.

HRCT is usually not required to monitor progress and response to treatment as chest radiograph alone is adequate for these purposes. In patients with prolonged illness and who are non-responsive to standard treatment, HRCT may help to assess pulmonary parenchymal abnormalities — to ascertain whether the predominant component is ground-glass opacification (which is considered to be reversible and amenable to medical treatment) or fibrosis (which is considered as irreversible lung damage).

CLINICO-RADIOLOGICAL CORRELATION — PROGNOSTIC INDICATORS

The extent of pneumonia on the presentation chest radiograph appears to correlate with adverse clinical outcome in SARS. Those who either require ICU care or die have more extensive radiological evidence of pneumonia on the initial CXR. These patients with poor outcome have a

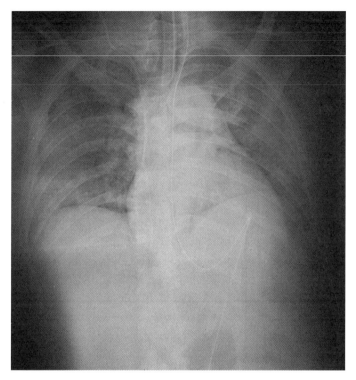

Fig. 10 Frontal chest radiograph in a 30-year-old SARS patient shows confluent air-space opacification in both lungs compatible with changes of acute respiratory distress syndrome (ARDS).

worse chest radiograph compared with those with better prognosis at presentation and at day 7 after fever onset. Patients with consolidation > 1 zone on the initial CXR and day 7 CXR, are more likely to progress to ICU admission/death than those with ≤ 1 zone involvement.

Patients with bilateral pneumonic changes on the initial CXR are more likely to require ICU care or have a fatal outcome in comparison with those with unilateral pneumonia on admission. Multivariable analysis has shown that more than one CXR zone involvement on presentation is an independent predictor of an adverse outcome after adjustment is made for high baseline LDH, advanced age and a high neutrophil count.

In our experience, the pattern of radiographic progression correlates well with clinical outcome.[3] In patients with Type 1 pattern on serial CXR, only 17.5% are either admitted to ICU or dead, whereas 51.2% with CXR category other than Type 1 are either admitted to ICU or dead. Patients with Type 1 pattern (initial radiographic progression followed by improvement) on serial CXR have a more favorable outcome, whereas patients with Type 4 pattern (progressive deterioration) have an adverse clinical outcome.

Among all the laboratory parameters, there is a positive correlation between CXR trend and the rate of change of LDH, a marker of tissue damage. There is significant correlation between the rate of change of LDH (units/day) with the rate of change of radiographic involvement. LDH most likely reflects the extent of lung injury in this setting.

FOLLOW-UP

After treatment for SARS and discharge from hospital, some patients complain of exertional dyspnea and reduced exercise tolerance. Residual CXR abnormalities are present in some patients and HRCT helps to accurately depict the underlying lung parenchymal abnormality. Preliminary observations show that more than 90% of these symptomatic patients have residual ground-glass opacification[14] (Fig. 11). About 60% of these patients have evidence of probable fibrosis (presence of parenchymal

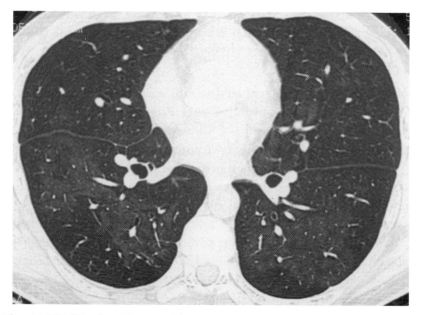

Fig. 11 HRCT of a 37-year-old SARS patient 2 months after discharge shows residual ground-glass opacification in both lower lobes.

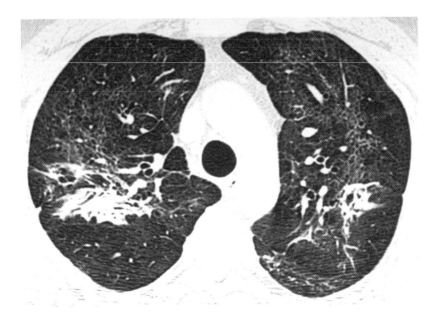

Fig. 12 HRCT of a 39-year-old SARS patient 6 weeks after discharge shows conglomerate fibrosis with architectural distortion involving both upper lobes. Residual ground-glass opacification are present in the rest of both upper lobes.

bands, irregular surface and traction bronchiectasis) on follow-up HRCT after discharge[14] (Fig. 12). Patients with evidence of probable fibrosis at one month follow-up are older and have more severe disease during the period of treatment (higher intensive admission rate, more steroid dosage required, higher peak LDH level and higher peak CXR changes) than those without such HRCT changes.

Although the HRCTs after discharge do show evidence of residual disease and probable fibrotic change, follow-up imaging at six months correlated with clinical parameters (including lung function test) would be more accurate in reflecting the true extent of permanent lung damage and its implication on the patients' daily activities and exercise tolerance.

INFECTION CONTROL MEASURES IN RADIOLOGY DEPARTMENT

In the face of this highly infectious disease, it is important to reduce the risk of cross infection between patients as well as reducing the risk of infection to staff. With close collaboration with the hospital infection control team, certain procedures and guidelines must be implemented to ensure stringent infection control within the Radiology Department. These include:

- Physical segregation of patients with suspected or confirmed SARS by allocating portable radiographic equipment in a different location outside the main Radiology Department.
- For imaging modalities with equipment/machine which cannot be moved away from the main Radiology Department (eg CT scanner), segregation of patients is achieved by allocating a separate period for scanning of suspected or confirmed SARS patients.
- Staff education to ensure various infection control measures are strictly adhered to.

REFERENCES

1. World Health Organization. Case definition of severe acute respiratory syndrome (SARS). (Available at http://www.who.int/csr/sars/casedefinition/en/. Accessed 20 May 2003).

2. Centre for Disease Control and Prevention, USA. Diagnosis/evaluation for SARS. (Accessed April 7, 2003, at http://www.cdc.gov/ncidod/sars/diagnosis.htm).

3. Wong KT, Antonio GE, Hui DS, *et al.* Severe acute respiratory syndrome: Radiographic appearances and pattern of progression in 138 patients. *Radiology*. 2003;**228**:401–406.

4. Wong KT, Antonio GE, Hui DS, *et al.* Thin-section CT of severe acute respiratory syndrome: Evaluation of 74 patients exposed to or with the disease. *Radiology*. 2003;**228**:395–400.

5. Antonio GE, Wong KT, Hui DS, *et al.* Imaging of severe acute respiratory syndrome in Hong Kong. *Am J Roentgenol* 2003;**181**:11–17.

6. Goodman LR, Goren RA, Teptick SK. The radiographic evaluation of pulmonary infection. *Med Clin North Am* 1980;**64**(3):553–74.

7. Macfarlane JT, Miller AC, Roderick Smith WH, *et al.* Comparative radiographic features of community acquired Legionnaires disease, pneumococcal pneumonia, mycoplasma pneumonia, and psittacosis. *Thorax* 1984;**39**(1):28–33.

8. Tanaka N, Matsumoto T, Kuramitsu T, *et al.* High resolution CT findings in community-acquired pneumonia. *J Comput Assist Tomogr* 1996;**20**:600–608.

9. John SD, Ramanathan J, Swischuk LE. Spectrum of clinical and radiographic findings in pediatric mycoplasma pneumonia. *Radiographics* 2001;**21**(1):121–31.

10. Reittner P, Muller NL, Heyneman L, *et al.* Mycoplasma pneumoniae pneumonia: Radiographic and high-resolution CT features in 28 patients. *Am J Roentgenol* 2000;**174**:37–41.

11. Kim EA, Lee KS, Primack SL, *et al.* Viral pneumonias in adults: Radiologic and pathologic findings. *Radiographics* 2002;**22**(suppl): 137S–149S.

12. Lee N, Hui D, Wu A, *et al.* A major outbreak of severe acute respiratory syndrome in Hong Kong. *N Engl J Med* 2003;**348**(20):1986–94.

13. Peiris JS, Chu CM, Cheng VC, *et al.* Clinical progression and viral load in a community outbreak of coronavirus-associated SARS pneumonia: A prospective study. *Lancet* 2003;**361**:1767–1772.

14. Antonio GE, Wong KT, Hui DS, *et al.* Thin-section computed tomography in patients with severe acute respiratory syndrome following hospital discharge: Preliminary experience. *Radiology* 2003;**228**:810–815.

9

Hematology and Immunology

Raymond SM Wong, Gregory Cheng

INTRODUCTION

Infection with the SARS-coronavirus produces changes in various organ systems in addition to lung injury. Immune-mediated mechanisms have been proposed as playing an important role in the progress of SARS. This chapter summarizes the hematological manifestations of SARS, the immunological changes associated with it, and our experience with the use of convalescent plasma therapy to manage the disease.

HEMATOLOGICAL CHANGES IN PATIENTS WITH SEVERE ACUTE RESPIRATORY SYNDROME

Viral infection may produce a variety of hematological changes. The hematological findings reported here are based on a cohort of 157 patients with SARS as confirmed by serological study (and who had no pre-existing hematological disorder) treated at the Prince of Wales Hospital, Hong Kong.[1] The cohort included 64 males and 93 females and all were ethnically Chinese. The mean age was 38.5 years (range, 20 to 83 years) and the median duration of follow-up was 26 days (range, 4 to 38 days). All the patients received broad-spectrum antibiotics, and a combination of ribavirin and prednisolone 0.5 mg/kg/day as empirical therapy. Intravenous high-dose methylprednisolone was used in patients with respiratory distress or progressive consolidations on chest radiograph.

White Blood Cell Disorders

Leukocyte disorders may show considerable variations in the different viral infections and result in numerical, morphologic, immunologic and functional abnormalities. During the first week of illness, transient leucopenia (leukocyte count, $<4 \times 10^9/L$) was detected in 64% of the patients. As their diseases progressed, leucocyte count gradually recovered in the majority of the patients, with about 60% of them developing leucocytosis (leukocyte count, $>11 \times 10^9/L$) mostly in the second and third week of illness.

Neutrophils

Neutropenia (absolute neutrophil count (ANC), $<0.5 \times 10^9/L$) is a rare finding and usually last for 1–2 days. Neutrophilia (ANC, $>7.5 \times 10^9/L$) has been noted in about 80% of patients during their illness. A high neutrophil count at presentation has also been shown to be an independent predictor of death or admission to an intensive care unit.[2] While neutrophilia during the course of illness may be caused by demargination of neutrophils related to the use of corticosteroids, neutrophilia at any time was associated with a higher incidence of bacterial infections as documented by microbiological cultures. Most of these infections were hospital acquired pneumonia or line sepsis. In patients with neutrophilia, full sepsis work-up and empirical broad-spectrum antibiotics should be considered. The other possible reason for neutrophilia, especially on hospital admission, is tissue necrosis as a result of the viral infection.

Lymphocytes

Lymphopenia (absolute lymphocyte count, $<1000/mm^3$) is the most common finding in patients with SARS and has been found in about 98% of patients during their course of illness. A typical profile of change in lymphocyte count is shown in Fig. 1. The majority of patients had normal lymphocyte count at disease onset. Progressive lymphopenia occurred early in the course of illness and reached a nadir at the second week in most cases (Fig. 2). Recovery of lymphocyte count commonly occurs in the third week but about one-third of patients remain lymphopenic at the fifth week of SARS. Patients with more severe illness and prolonged respiratory distress show persistent lymphopenia and delay recovery of lymphocyte count.

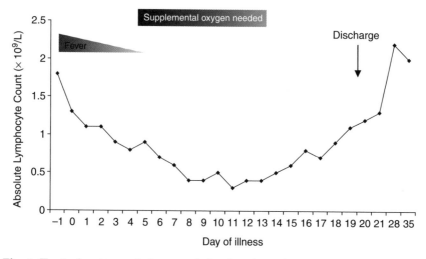

Fig. 1 Typical pattern of change of absolute lymphocyte count in patients with SARS.

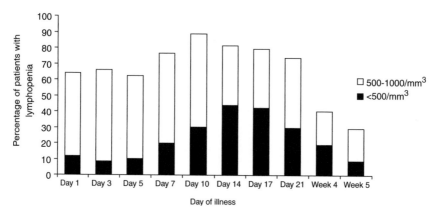

Fig. 2 Percentage of patients with absolute lymphopenia during the course of SARS.

In the Prince of Wales Hospital, analysis of peripheral blood lympho-cyte subsets was performed in a cohort of 31 patients. The mean CD4+ and CD8+ cell counts at presentation were 286.7 ± 142.2 cells/μL (reference range, 410 to 1590 cells/μL) and 242.2 ± 130.8 cells/μL (reference range, 190 to 1140 cells/μL) respectively (Fig. 3). The number of CD3+, T-helper (CD4+) and T-suppressor (CD8+) lymphocytes respectively, decreased significantly early in the course of illness. The CD4/CD8 ratio remained stable. The natural killer cells also decreased significantly on day 4. The mean B-lymphocyte count in peripheral blood at presentation was 151.3 ± 73.2 per μL (reference range, 90–660 cells/μL) and it remained sta-ble. Low CD4 and CD8 counts at presentation were found to be associated with death or admission to an intensive care unit. The patients in this sub-group were young (median age 27 years, range 21 to 58 years) with no comorbidity. The low CD4+ and CD8+ cell counts likely reflected the severity of the illness and are therefore good markers of disease activity. In another study, Tang *et al.* also reported similar changes of T-lymphocytes, which were different from the observations in patients with AIDS who had decreased CD4+ but increased CD8+ lymphocytes.[3] These changes in T-lymphocytes are reversible and the recovery of the T-lymphocytes is sig-nificantly faster in the mild cases than in the severe cases.[4]

Post-mortem examination demonstrated lymphopenia in various lymphoid organs. No enlarged lymph nodes were seen in the peripheral soft tissues or other body parts and no reactive lymphoid hyperplasia was noted. Reactive lymphoid follicular hyperplasia or T zone reaction was not seen (Fig. 4a). The spleens were not enlarged and splenic white pulps appeared atrophic with lymphoid depletion, and the red pulp was congested (Fig. 4b). Bone marrow appeared active with presentation of trilineage hematopoiesis (Fig. 4c) but with no feature of reactive hemopagocytic syndrome was noted. The pulmonary pathology of the fatal cases was dominated by diffuse alveolar damage and the lymphoid infiltrate was spares.

Depletion of lymphocytes may be secondary to the direct effect of virus on the lymphocytes or the effect of various cytokines.[5,6] Gu *et al.* demonstrated that the immune cells, particularly T lymphocytes, har-bored a large amount of SARS coronavirus particles in their cytoplasm.[7] Most of the circulating lymphocytes were infected by the virus. About 20% of the lymphocytes in the spleen and lymph nodes were positive for SARS coronavirus by in-situ hybridization. It appears that the

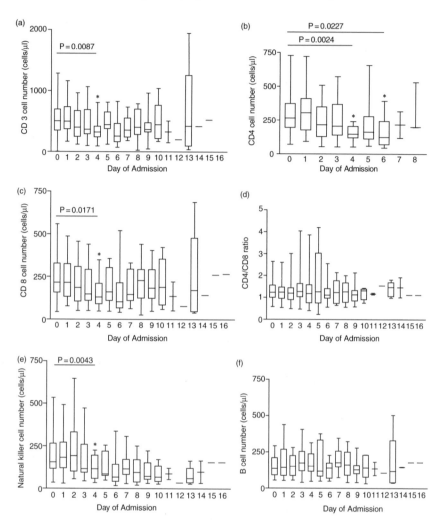

Fig. 3 Change of (a) CD3+ lymphocytes; (b) CD4+ lymphocytes; (c) CD8+ lymphocytes; (d) CD4/CD8 ratio; (e) natural killer cells; and (f) B lymphocytes in peripheral blood during the course of illness in 31 patients with SARS. (Courtesy of Dr. CK Wong and Professor CWK Lam, Department of Chemical Pathology, Chinese University of Hong Kong.)

coronavirus causing SARS is lymphotrophic and lymphotoxic, but the underlying mechanisms remain obscure. The damage of cellular immunity may be an important mechanism of pathogenesis of SARS. Further study of the mechanism of entry of coronavirus into the T-lymphocytes

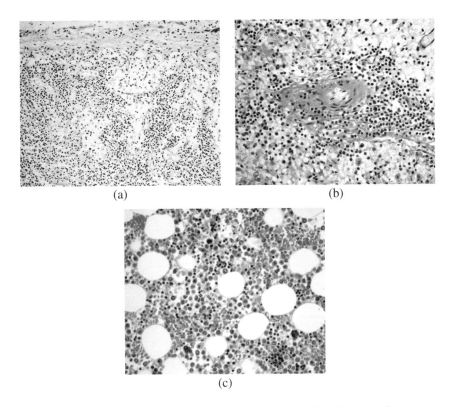

(a)

(b)

(c)

Fig. 4 (a) Lymph node histology. No reactive lymphoid hyperplasia was noted. Mild dialation of the lymph node sinuses was noted in this lymph node. No features of reactive hemopagocytic syndrome were noted (H&E stain, X100). (b) Spleen. White pulp depletion was noted. Only scanty amount of lymphoid cells were surrounding the splenic arterioles (H&E stain, X200). (c) Bone marrow. The bone marrow appeared active and trilineage hematopoiesis was presented (H&E stain, X200). (Courtesy of Dr. KF To, Department of Anatomical & Cellular Pathology, Chinese University of Hong Kong.)

and the subsequent alteration in the cellular immunity may help to develop more effective treatment strategies and reduce the complications of SARS.

Platelet

Thrombocytopenia followed by reactive thrombocytosis is another common finding in patients with SARS. In the Prince of Wales Hospital cohorts, about 55% of the patients developed thrombocytopenia (platelet

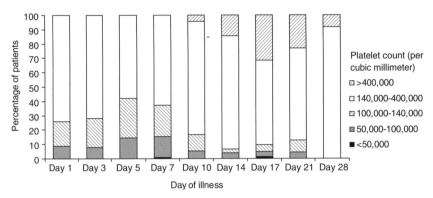

Fig. 5 Percentage of patients with various levels of platelet counts during the course of SARS.

count, $<140,000/\text{mm}^3$) during their course of illness (Fig. 5). Most of the patients had normal platelet count at presentation and progressive thrombocytopenia occurred as the disease progressed and reached a nadir at the end of the first week. The majority of them had mild thrombocytopenia (platelet count $50–140,000/\text{mm}^3$) and only 2% of them had platelet count less than $50,000/\text{mm}^3$ (Fig. 5). Thrombocytopenia is usually self-limiting and resolves by the fourth week of illness. Few patients had major bleeding or requiring platelet transfusion. Thrombocytopenia has been reported in many viral infection.[8–13] It may be caused by immune destruction or the direct effect of viruses on megakaryocytes or platelets.[8] Megakaryocytes may harbor a variety of viruses, although the mechanism of viral entry into megakaryocytes is not certain. Infected megakaryocytes may show dysmorphic features such as inclusion bodies, vacuoles, degenerating nuclei, or naked nuclei.[14] In the Prince of Wales Hospital cohort, there was no evidence of frank DIC in the majority of the cases. The autopsy findings of active bone marrow with normal megakaryoctes in the fatal cases with thrombocytopenia suggest an immune cause of thrombocytopenia.

Reactive thrombocytosis (platelet count, $>400,000/\text{mm}^3$) was noted in about half of the patients (Fig. 6). The platelet count reached a peak on a median 17 days after onset of the illness (range, day 6 to 31). Only one patient had platelet count above $1\,000\,000/\text{mm}^3$. Micro-emboli were found in post-mortem cases but the significance is unsure. Clinical thrombotic complications have not been documented.

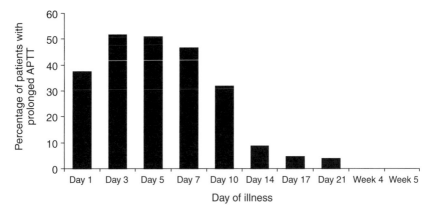

Fig. 6 Percentage of patients with abnormal APTT during the course of SARS.

Hemoglobin

A major side effect of ribavirin is reversible hemolytic anemia.[15,16] In the Prince of Wales Hospital cohort, about 60% of the patients showed a drop in hemoglobin of more than 20 g/L from baseline, and nearly 30% of the patients experienced a drop of hemoglobin of more than 30 g/L after a two-week course of ribavirin, at a dose of 400 mg every 8 hours intravenously or 1200 mg thrice daily orally. There was no evidence of major bleeding in all the patients. Despite such a high incidence of hemoglobin drop, ribavirin was well tolerated and none of them required withdrawal of treatment or transfusion. Of the patients with a hemoglobin drop of more than 20 g/L, 60% of the patients showed evidence of hemolysis (rise of bilirubin >20 μmol/L and/or reticulocyte count >1%). Direct and indirect Coomb's tests showed no evidence of immune cause of hemolysis. Hemolysis was transient and hemoglobin level gradually recovered after completion of ribavirin treatment in all the patients. Careful monitoring of hemoglobin is advisable for patients treated with ribavirin.

Clotting Profile

Isolated prolonged activated partial thromboplastin time (APTT) is another common hematological finding in patients with SARS. About

63% of the patients in the Prince of Wales Hospital group developed isolated prolonged APTT (>40 seconds). Their APTT results ranged from 40 to 68 seconds and occurred mainly in the first two weeks of illness. There was no evidence of venous thromboembolism or other coagulation abnormalities such as the presence of the anti-cardiolipin antibody or grossly elevated D-dimer levels. The D-dimer levels were normal in most of the cases and mildly raised (500–1000 ng/L) in some cases. None of the patients required plasma transfusion or treatment with clotting factors. The abnormal clotting profile was self-limiting and all the patients had normal APTT at week 4. About one-third of the patients had no abnormality in clotting profile throughout their course of illness.

A few patients (2.5%) developed frank disseminated intravascular coagulation (DIC) with prolonged PT, APTT, thrombocytopenia and elevated D-dimer levels. All of them had severe illness at the time of DIC and eventually died of severe respiratory distress with multi-organ failure with or without superimposed bacterial infections. Some of the patients also showed a mildly raised level of D-dimer in the range of 500–1000 ng/L with normal clotting profile. Hemorrhagic-fever-like illness with laboratory evidence of mild DIC has also been reported in one case.[17]

TREATMENT OF SARS USING PASSIVE IMMUNIZATION WITH CONVALESCENT PLASMA

As of June 2003, there were over 8000 cases of SARS worldwide, with more than 600 deaths. Treatment has been empirical and there is no general consensus on treatment. In Hong Kong, ribavirin and steroids were used as first line treatment to suppress viral replication and minimize autoimmune pneumonitis. The ribavirin-steroid combination was associated with favorable recovery in about three quarters of the patients. However, those patients with persistent fever, radiographic progression and hypoxemia after three days of methylprednisolone, usually responded poorly to a further course of high dose steroid. Many of them required admission to an intensive care unit, mechanical ventilation and had a high mortality rate. We anticipated that the convalescent plasma of SARS patients would carry antibodies against coronavirus and may suppress viremia. We report here our experience with convalescent plasma therapy in patients who failed to respond to ribavirin and high dose steroid therapy.

USE OF CONVALESCENT PLASMA IN VIRAL DISEASES

Treatment of viral disease using convalescent plasma/serum has a long history dating back to the nineteenth century. In 1891, a young girl with diphtheria received a sheep antiserum against the diphtheria toxin and recovered within hours. Clinical benefits of convalescent plasma therapy were observed in the Machupo virus Bolivain haemorrhagic fever epidemic in 1960,[18] the Junin virus Argentina hemorrhagic fever epidemic[19] and the Lassa fever epidemic in Nigeria in the 1980's.[20] The mortality rate in 448 patients with the Argentine fever before the convalescent plasma era was 43%. From 1959 to 1983, 4433 patients with Argentine hemorrhagic fever was treated using convalescent plasma, and the overall mortality was 3.29%. Twenty-seven patients with suspected or diagnosed Lassa fever in Nigeria were treated with convalescent plasma. Fifteen patients received convalescent plasma on or before day 10 of the illness, and all of them recovered and survived. On the other hand, only four out of the eight patients who received plasma after day 10 survived. In June 1995, eight patients in the Democratic Republic of Congo with severe Ebola virus hemorrhagic fever were transfused with 150–450 ml of convalescent blood from recovered patients. Seven patients survived, as compared with a case fatality rate of over 80 percent in many Ebola virus patients.[21] West Nile encephalitis is an emerging viral disease in the United States. It is a mosquito-borne disease that can rapidly progress to meningitis or encephalitis in humans. Pooled plasma or immunoglobulin from recovered patients had full protective effects in infected mice and clinical benefits in patients.[22,23]

THE PRINCE OF WALES HOSPITAL EXPERIENCE

At the Prince of Wales Hospital, convalescent plasma was obtained from patients who recovered from SARS (informed consent given), using a Baxter CS 300 cell separator. The donor must be afebrile for at least 7 consecutive days, had radiographic improvement of over 25%, had no further need of oxygen supplement and at least 14 days had passed since symptoms onset. The donors must also be hepatitis B, C, HIV and VDRL seronegative. All the plasma donors had a coronavirus titre of 160–2560 at the time of plasma collection. The blood volume processed ranged from

2000 to 2500 ml. An average of 600 to 1000 ml of plasma was harvested from each donor and stored as 200 ml aliquots. The patients each received 200–400 ml of ABO compatible plasma. Between 10 March to 10 April 2003, 40 patients had progressive disease after 3 doses (500 mg each) of pulsed methylprednisolone. Nineteen of the patients were given convalescent plasma and 21 patients were given further four to eight doses of pulsed methylprednisolone. There were no differences in age, sex and admission LDH between the two groups (Table 1). No immediate adverse effects were observed with convalescent plasma infusion. 74% of the patients in the plasma group were discharged by day 22 as compared with 19% in the steroid group ($p = 0.001$). There were 5 deaths in the steroid group, as compared with zero death in the plasma group ($p < 0.001$). Since then, we had treated a further 50 patients with convalescent plasma. Thirty-three patients received convalescent serum before day 16 of onset of the illness. Of these, 16 (48%) had good clinical outcomes. Seventeen patients received convalescent plasma after day 16, and none was discharged at day 22 ($p = 0.001$, Table 2). The death rates in the two groups were 3% and 29.4% respectively ($p = 0.014$). In general,

Table 1 Clinical Characteristics and Treatment Outcome of the Plasma and Steroid Group

	Plasma Group (3 MP + CP)	Steroid Group (4 or more MP)	p Value
No. of patients	19	21	
Age	38.7 ± 12.39	47.9 ± 19.60	0.087
Admission lactate dehydrogenase level (IU/L)	256.1 ± 90.75	247.7 ± 94.58	0.7
Discharge rate by day 22 of onset of illness	73.4% ($n = 14$)	19% ($n = 4$)	0.001
Death rate	0%	23.8% ($n = 5$)	0.049

MP indicates methylprednisolone; CP, convalescent plasma

Table 2 Outcomes of Patients Given Convalescent Plasma before Day 16 versus Those Given after Day 16

	≤Day 16	>Day 16	p Values
Discharge rate by day 22	48% ($n = 16$)	0% ($n = 0$)	0.0001
Death rate	3% ($n = 1$)	29.4% ($n = 5$)	0.014

patients with good clinical outcomes had been given convalescent plasma much earlier than the poor outcome group (11.9 vs. 15.8 days, $p = 0.002$). These preliminary data showed that patients who deteriorated despite ribavirin and high dose steroid had a more favorable outcome when given convalescent plasma, as compared with those continuing on high dose methylprednisolone without convalescent plasma.

POSSIBLE MECHANISMS OF CONVALESCENT PLASMA IN SARS

In SARS, the viral load peaks around day 10 and starts to decline as coronavirus specific antibodies started to appear. Clinical deterioration in the third week is thought to be the result of inflammatory or hyper immune attacks on lung tissues. It has been clearly demonstrated with electronic microscopy that coronavirus were present in peripheral blood lymphocytes, lymph nodes, spleen, brain tissues and lung tissues. Lymphopenia may be the result of direct cytopathic effects of the virus and clinical recovery is usually associated with recovery of lymphocytes counts. Reducing the viral load in the first two weeks may reduce the direct viral induced damage and the subsequent immune mediated damage in the third week, thereby improving clinical outcomes. In Lassa fever, patients treated with convalescent plasma on or before day 10 of the illness had a much higher survival rate compared with those given convalescent plasma after day 10.[20] Our observation that convalescent plasma is more effective when given before day 16 is consistent with the above hypothesis.

FUTURE DIRECTIONS OF DEVELOPMENT

Our study had several limitations. First of all, it was not a randomized study. Whether the patient received convalescent plasma or steroids depended on the physician's preference and the availability of convalescent plasma. A larger randomized study is required to confirm our observation and determine the most appropriate timing and dosage of convalescent plasma. Secondly, the amount of coronavirus specific antibodies given to each patient was not standardized. In Lassa fever, the efficacy of passive immunization with convalescent plasma is also believed to depend on the titer of the neutralizing antibodies infused.[24] Accurate quantitative assays of coronavirus neutralizing antibodies are now being developed; this will improve standardization of convalescent plasma therapy in SARS. Finally, even though we have not observed any anaphylactic reaction or immediate adverse effects with plasma infusion, the risk of transfusion transmitted infection cannot be excluded. Ideally, convalescent plasma should be treated with an effective viral inactivation procedure before infusion into recipients. Our preliminary study in SARS and worldwide experience of convalescent plasma therapy in other viral epidemics suggested a role of viral inactivated convalescent plasma or coronavirus-specific hyperimmunoglobulin in future outbreaks.

SUMMARY

Lymphopenia, in particular T-lymphopenia, is common in patients with SARS. A significant drop in CD4+ and CD8+ lymphocytes occurs early in the course of SARS and is associated with adverse outcomes. The damage in cellular immunity may play an important role in the pathogenesis and progress of SARS. Thrombocytopenia, neutrophilia and transient prolonged APTT are other common hematological findings. Further studies to evaluate the mechanisms of the change in the immune system may help to develop more effective therapeutic options. Our data also suggests that convalescent plasma may be beneficial to patients with SARS before an active anti-viral agent can be identified.

REFERENCES

1. Wong RS, Wu A, To KF, *et al*. Haematological manifestations in patients with severe acute respiratory syndrome: Retrospective analysis. *BMJ* 2003;**326**:1358–62.

2. Lee N, Hui D, Wu A, *et al*. A major outbreak of severe acute respiratory syndrome in Hong Kong. *N Engl J Med* 2003;**348**:1986–94.

3. Tang X, Yin C, Zhang F, *et al*. Measurement of subgroups of peripheral blood T lymphocytes in patients with severe acute respiratory syndrome and its clinical significance. *Chin Med J (Engl)* 2003; **116**:827–30.

4. Liu S, Dai W, Zhang JW, Feng X. Changes of peripheral blood T lymphocytes in patients with severe acute respiratory syndrome. In *2003 International Symposium on Pathogenesis of SARS*. 2003. Beijing, China.

5. Maury CP and Lahdevirta J. Correlation of serum cytokine levels with haematological abnormalities in human immunodeficiency virus infection. *J Intern Med* 1990;**227**:253–7.

6. Van Campen H, Easterday BC, Hinshaw VS. Destruction of lymphocytes by a virulent avian influenza A virus. *J Gen Virol* 1989;**70** (Pt 2):467–72.

7. Gu J, Team SPR. The Pathogenetic Mechanisms of SARS. In *2003 International Symposium on Pathogenesis of SARS*. 2003. Beijing, China.

8. Zucker-Franklin D. The effect of viral infections on platelets and megakaryocytes. *Semin Hematol* 1994;**31**:329–37.

9. Eisenberg MJ, Kaplan B. Cytomegalovirus-induced thrombocytopenia in an immunocompetent adult. *West J Med* 1993;**158**:525–6.

10. Ninomiya N, Maeda T, Matsuda I. Thrombocytopenic purpura occurring during the early phase of a mumps infection. *Helv Paediatr Acta* 1977;**32**:87–9.

11. Oski FA, Naiman, JL. Effect of live measles vaccine on the platelet count. *N Engl J Med* 1966;**275**:352–6.

12. van Spronsen, DJ Breed, WP. Cytomegalovirus-induced thrombocytopenia and haemolysis in an immunocompetent adult. *Br J Haematol* 1996;**92**:218–20.

13. Ballem PJ, Belzberg A, Devine DV, *et al*. Kinetic studies of the mechanism of thrombocytopenia in patients with human immunodeficiency virus infection. *N Engl J Med* 1992;**327**:1779–84.

14. Chesney PJ, Taher A, Gilbert EM, Shahidi NT. Intranuclear inclusions in megakaryocytes in congenital cytomegalovirus infection. *J Pediatr* 1978;**92**:957–8.

15. McCromick JB, King IJ, Webb PA, *et al*. Lassa fever. Effective therapy with ribavirin. *N Engl J Med* 1986;**314**:20–26.

16. Roberts RB, Laskin OL, KLaurence J, *et al*. Ribavirin pharmacodynamics in high-risk patients for acquired immunodeficiency syndrome. *Clin Pharmacol Ther* 1987;**42**:365–373.

17. Wu EB, Sung JJ. Haemorrhagic-fever-like changes and normal chest radiograph in a doctor with SARS. *Lancet* 2003;**361**:1520–1.

18. Stinebaugh BJ, Schloeder FX, Johnson KM, *et al*. Bolivian hemorrhagic fever. A report of four cases. *Am J Med* 1966;**40**:217–30.

19. Ruggiero HA, Perez Isquierdo F, Milani HA, *et al*. Treatment of Argentine hemorrhagic fever with convalescent's plasma. 4433 cases. *Presse Med* 1986;**15**:2239–42.

20. Frame JD, Verbrugge GP, Gill RG, Pinneo L. The use of Lassa fever convalescent plasma in Nigeria. *Trans R Soc Trop Med Hyg* 1984; **78**:319–24.

21. Mupapa K, Massamba M, Kibadi K, *et al*. Treatment of Ebola hemorrhagic fever with blood transfusions from convalescent patients. International Scientific and Technical Committee. *J Infect Dis* 1999;**179** Suppl 1:S18–23.

22. Solomon T, Ooi MH, Beasley DW, Mallewa M. West Nile encephalitis. *Br Med J* 2003;**326**:865–9.

23. Ben-Nathan D, Lustig S, Tam G, *et al*. Prophylactic and therapeutic efficacy of human intravenous immunoglobulin in treating West Nile virus infection in mice. *J Infect Dis* 2003;**188**:5–12.

24. Jahrling PB, Frame JD, Rhoderick JB, *et al*. Lassa fever in Liberia. IV. Selection of optimally effective plasma for treatment by passive immunization. *Trans R Soc Trop Med Hyg* 1985;**79**:380–4.

10

The Medical Management of Severe Acute Respiratory Syndrome

JJY Sung, AKL Wu

INTRODUCTION

In March 2003, there was an outbreak of a new infectious disease worldwide, now known as the Severe Acute Respiratory Syndrome (SARS). A novel coronavirus has been shown in animal experiments to fulfill Koch's postulates and is now unequivocally identified as the causative agent for this new disease syndrome.[1] Thus far, published research data related to SARS generally converge on two areas: (1) the biology of the coronavirus, through the identification of its basic biochemical and genomic characteristics;[2–7] and (2) the clinical features of SARS through the description of the natural history, symptomatology and radiologic findings associated with the disease.[8–13] Despite the extensive amount of research done globally, relatively little information so far has been available regarding the optimal management of patients diagnosed with SARS. This is perhaps a bit surprising given the substantial morbidity and mortality of the disease. Clearly, much more active and organized research is urgently required in this particular area in order to resolve the many controversies that the practicing clinicians are now facing.

GENERAL MANAGEMENT OF SARS PATIENTS

At present, the most efficacious treatment regime for SARS is still not known. There is no formal treatment recommended except for meticulous supportive care. The following information is adapted from the guidelines published by the World Health Organization (WHO) (updated April 11). The reader is encouraged to check the Center for Disease Control (CDC) and WHO websites regularly for new updates:

http://www.who.int/csr/sars/management/en/

http://www.cdc.gov/ncidod/sars/treatment.htm

All patients fulfilling the case definitions for suspected or probable SARS who need to be admitted to hospitals should be placed under isolation or cohorted with other similar cases. Various samples (including sputum, blood, sera, urine) should be taken to exclude other causes of pneumonia (including those caused by atypical pathogens); appropriate chest radiographs should also be taken. Clinicians should always bear in mind the possibility of co-infection with SARS in patients who are thought to have other causes for their pneumonia.

Initial investigations for these patients should include complete blood counts, total white cell counts with differentials, platelet counts, urea and electrolytes, creatine phosphokinase, liver function tests, C reactive protein and paired sera samples (acute and convalescent, the latter to be taken >22–28 days after symptoms onset) for SARS-associated coronavirus (SARS-CoV), as well as for other conventional bacterial or viral pathogens. Respiratory samples, urine, plasma and stool samples should be taken for appropriate diagnostic evaluation of SARS-CoV (reverse transcriptase polymerase chain reactions and virus isolations using Vero cell cultures).

At the time of admission, the use of antibiotics for the treatment of community-acquired pneumonia with atypical cover is recommended (i.e. a third generation cephalosporin plus a macrolide , or a quinolone). Particular attention should be paid to therapies or interventions that may cause aerolization such as the use of nebulizers, chest physiotherapy, endoscopies, as well as any procedure or intervention that may cause disruption to the respiratory tract. Appropriate precautions should be taken (isolation facility, gloves, goggles, mask, gown, etc.) if such procedures are deemed necessary. The use of specific anti-viral and immunomodulatory therapies directed against the SARS-CoV, such as ribavirin and corticosteroids, will be discussed in greater detail in the following sections.

For patients with SARS who deteriorate despite treatment and require mechanical ventilation, they should be managed in intensive care units. Treatment is mainly supportive, although novel salvage therapies may also be considered (details given in the following sections). Most of these patients have diffuse infiltrates on chest radiography and hypoxemia, a condition known as adult respiratory distress syndrome (ARDS). The best approach for ventilatory support of patients at this stage is not known but should probably follow a lung-protective approach.[14]

A patient may be considered for discharge from hospital if he or she has been afebrile for 48 hours with clinical improvement, associated with normalization of abnormal laboratory parameters and resolving radiographic opacities. Convalescent patients should stay at home and avoid contacts with others for a minimum of one week following discharge, and they should monitor their own body temperatures at home. Convalescent patients should take enteric, droplets and contact precautions while they are at home during the early post-discharge period. They should be reviewed in clinics one week after discharge with repeat chest radiography and blood tests.

SPECIFIC TREATMENT REGIME FOR SARS

1. Pathogenesis of disease and general treatment principles

Before going into the various treatment regimes, it is useful to have a brief review of the pathogenesis of SARS. The following section contains material adapted from the Hong Kong Hospital Authority SARS management guidelines (updated May 15, accessed online at: http://www.ha.org.hk/sars/ps/information/treatment.htm), as well as information from experts in the field. Interested readers are encouraged to check the website for the latest guidelines.

Based on the clinical courses of over 270 patients, and serial measurements of viral load of coronavirus in some of these patients, SARS can be represented as a triphasic disease.[15,16]

In the first week of the illness, most patients presented with fever, myalgia and chills, with or without diarrhea, thrombocytopenia, lymphopenia, and liver dysfunction. There is usually no or minimal respiratory symptoms, with static or slow progression of radiographic opacities. This is the early or first phase when viral replication is most severe, and the virus itself is causing detrimental effects on the host. The disease progresses relatively slowly and some patients may spontaneously improve at this stage. At least 70% of patients then proceed to the second phase, which usually occurs in the second week of illness. During this phase of the disease, early response cytokines such as TNFa, IL–1, IL–6 and IL–8 are produced in large quantities, producing a so-called "cytokine storm" which contribute to immune dysregulation in the affected hosts. There is evidence of immunopathological damage to the lungs due to the mounting of host cell-mediated immune response. The patients start to develop typical respiratory symptoms, including shortness of breath (especially in the standing or sitting position), cough with pinkish sputum, while chest radiograph shows multiple areas of consolidation involving both lungs. There may be a resurgence of fever, and patients may suddenly deteriorate with marked desaturation. In the third week of disease, some patients may progress into the third phase of immunoparesis with severe respiratory failure and bilateral ground glass radiographic changes of ARDS. This is the third or pulmonary destruction phase of the disease. Histopathological examinations of autopsy cases reveal marked infiltration by macrophages, hemophagocytosis and hyaline membrane formation, consistent with the hypothesis of immune-mediated damage.[16] Eventually, a reasonable oxygenation saturation level cannot be maintained, and patients will require positive pressure ventilation. For reasons not entirely clear at this point, patients at this stage of the disease are more prone to develop barotraumas with spontaneous pneumothorax or pneumomediastinum, especially if they require invasive ventilation. Finally, concomitant hospital acquired sepsis and reactivation of latent infection may then set in and contribute substantially to patient morbidity and mortality.

Based on the proposed pathogenesis of SARS, the following general treatment strategy has been adopted in Hong Kong (see HA SARS treatment guidelines, updated 12 May 2003):

Phase 1 or viral replicative phase

Only antiviral agents, either in isolation or combined, should be used to suppress viral replication at this stage. The use of high-dose corticosteroids or other immunomodulating agents should, in general, be avoided at this stage. Examples of antivirals that have been used or proposed include ribavirin and protease inhibitors such as lopinavir-ritonavir (Kaletra™).

Phase 2 or immune hyperactive phase

Initiation of corticosteroid treatment according to the occurrence and severity of lung damage is currently recommended for management of this phase of the disease. The aim of the treatment is to reduce the incidence of respiratory failure and hence the need for ventilatory support (with the accompanying risk of subsequent nosocomial complications), and to limit the degree of residual lung damage.

Phase 3 or pulmonary destruction phase

For those patients who do not respond to corticosteroids, they should be given salvage immunomodulatory therapy, in order to limit the extent of the on-going immune-mediated pulmonary damage, and prevent the development of ARDS. Agents such as intravenous immunoglobulins and anti-cytokine therapy have been tried in this phase of the disease. No formal recommendations exist for the use of these agents up to the time of writing of this article, and their use should be regarded as experimental at this stage.

2. Management of SARS: the PWH experience

In March 2003, there was a major outbreak of SARS in Hong Kong. We have previously reported the clinical and radiographic features of the initial cohort of 138 SARS patients that was admitted to our hospital for management.[8] Briefly, there were 66 males and 72 females with a mean age (± 1 SD) of 39.3 ± 16.8 years. Length of time between onset of symptoms and hospital admission ranged from 0 to 11 days (median 3 days). Of these 138 cases, 132 cases were subsequently classified as laboratory confirmed SARS cases (124 cases had serological evidence indicating recent SARS-CoV infection, while eight patients had SARS-CoV isolated from clinical or post-mortem specimens); only two patients were found to have definitive negative convalescent serology to SARS-CoV. The SARS team at the Prince of Wales Hospital were responsible for developing the stepwise management protocol (see Fig. 1). Patients were treated for the

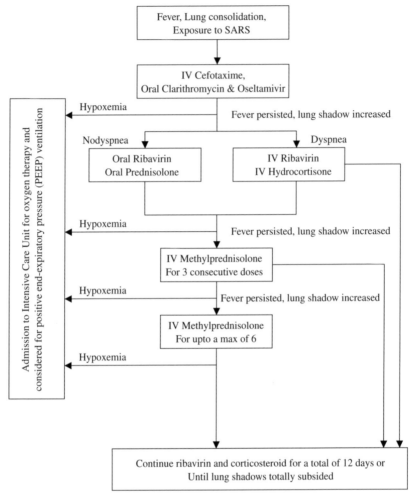

Fig. 1 Treatment Protocol for SARS in PWH.

first two days with broad-spectrum antibiotics for community-acquired pneumonia, according to the American Thoracic Society Guidelines.[18] Initial treatment consisted of intravenous cefotaxime 1 g every 6 hours and oral clarithromycin 500 mg twice daily (or oral levofloxacin 500 mg daily). Oseltamivir (Tamiflu™) was also given to some patients to treat possible influenza infection in the initial stages of the outbreak. If fever persisted, patients were given a combination of ribavirin and "low-dose" corticosteroid therapy commencing on day 3 or 4 (oral ribavirin as a loading dose of 2.4 g stat followed by 1.2 g three times daily and prednisolone

0.5–1 mg/kg body weight per day). Those with dyspnea at presentation were treated with intravenous ribavirin (400 mg every 8 hours) combined with hydrocortisone (100 mg every 8 hours). Pulses of high-dose methylprednisolone (0.5 g IVI for three consecutive days) were given as a response to persistence or recurrence of fever and radiographic progression of lung opacity ± hypoxemia despite initial combination therapy. Further pulses of methylprednisolone were given if there was no clinical or radiological improvement, up to a total of 3 grams.

Patients who developed hypoxemia were given supplemental oxygen therapy. Patients were admitted to the intensive care unit (ICU) when severe respiratory failure developed. Noninvasive positive pressure ventilation was avoided because of the potential risk of viral transmission. Patients were intubated and ventilated if they exhibited: (1) persistent failure to achieve arterial oxygen saturation of 90% while receiving 100% oxygen via a non-rebreathing mask; and/or (2) onset of respiratory muscle fatigue as evidenced by an increase in $PaCO_2$, sweating, tachycardia and/or a subjective feeling of exhaustion. Mechanical ventilation with synchronized intermittent mandatory ventilation (SIMV), or pressure control ventilation was instituted. Positive end expiratory pressure (PEEP) and inspired oxygen concentration was titrated to achieve an arterial saturation of 90–95%. Tidal volume was maintained at 6–8 ml/kg estimated body weight and plateau pressure maintained at 30 cmH$_2$O or less. $PaCO_2$ was allowed to rise provided the pH was greater than 7.15.[18] Patients unable to meet the above parameters were ventilated in the prone position.

We defined clinical response to treatment according to a set of clinical and radiological criteria. Sustained response (SR) to therapy was defined as: (1) Defervescence (daily peak temperature ≤ 37.5°C) for at least four consecutive days; (2) Radiological improvement of chest opacities of ≥ 25%; and (3) Oxygen independence (SaO$_2$ ≥ 95% on room air) on the fourth afebrile day. Patients with defervescence who achieved either resolution of lung consolidation or oxygen independence, but not both, were classified as showing a partial response (PR). Patients who fell short of criteria (2) and (3) above were classified as non-responders to therapy (NR).

The treatment outcome of this cohort of SARS patients was shown in Table 1. None of the 138 cases responded to antibiotics. Ninety-four patients received oral ribavirin and prednisolone. Among them, there were 14 sustained responders and nine partial responders. These 23 patients

Table 1 Clinical Response to Therapy in PWH SARS Cohort

	Board-spectrum Antimicrobial* (%) N = 138	Ribavirin + Corticosteroid# (%) N = 138	IV Methyl-prednisolone+ (%) N = 107
Sustained response	0 (0)	16 (11.6)	50 (46.7)
Partial response	0 (0)	9 (6.5)	45 (42.1)
No response	138 (100)	113 (81.9)	12 (11.2)

*Antimicrobials included cefotaxime and clarithromycin (or levofloxacin) plus oseltamivir.
#Ribavirin (oral or intravenous) plus oral prednisolone or intravenous hydrocortisone.
+Intravenous Methylprednisolone up to 3 g in total.

Clinical outcome definitions:
1. afebrile (daily peak temperature ≤37.5°C) for at least 4 consecutive days.
2. resolution of chest radiograph consolidation by .25% (comparing film of maximal consolidation and that on the 4th afebrile day).
3. oxygen independence (SaO$_2$≥ 95% on room air) on the 4th afebrile day.

Sustained response = 1 + 2 + 3
Partial response = 1 + 2 or 3
No response = 5 failure to fulfill criteria of sustained response or partial response.

were discharged uneventfully. Two patients died in the early phase of the disease before additional therapy could be offered. Forty-four patients received intravenous ribavirin and hydrocortisone and, among them, only two had a sustained response whereas four patients died. This combination therapy failed to show any appreciable response in the remaining 107 patients. Overall, 25 patients (18.1%) responded to ribavirin and "low-dose" corticosteroid therapy alone, while 107 patients showed no response and were given pulsed methylprednisolone. After three infusions of 0.5 g methylprednisolone, 45 patients (42.1%) showed a sustained response and recovered from the disease. Fifty-two patients (48.6%) demonstrated a partial response to the therapy. Among those with a partial response, 31 recovered and were discharged from hospital, one died, while 20 required further pulses of high-dose methylprednisolone. There were 10 non-responders, and among them one died. Among the partial responders and non-responders, 29 received further doses of intravenous methylprednisolone for up to 3 g in total. Sustained response was reported in five and partial response in 13. Eleven patients failed to show any response to > 3 pulses of high-dose methylprednisolone. Among them, six patients died, one remained in the ICU, and one remained on medical ward, while 3 were discharged from hospital. The overall success rate of high-dose methyl-prednisolone therapy was 88.8%. A total of 37 (26.8%) patients were admitted to ICU, and among them, 21 (15.2%) required endotracheal intubation and mechanical ventilation. Barotrauma was noted in 8 patients (21.6% of ICU admissions). Pneumomediastinum with subcutaneous surgical emphysema was seen in 3 cases and pneumothorax in 5. At 3 months after the onset of the SARS outbreak, 121 (87.7%) patients had been discharged, whereas 2 (1.4%) still remained in hospital. There were 15 deaths (mortality 10.9%). The majority of those who died had co-existing medical co-morbidities such as diabetes mellitus, chronic liver and cardiac diseases.

We also performed a multivariate analysis to determine the factors predicting the need for high dose methylprednisolone therapy (i.e. failure of ribavirin and low dose corticosteroid) in our cohort. A high presenting LDH level (Odds ratio per 100U/L, 1.56; 95 percent confidence interval 1.07, 2.25; $p = 0.02$) was found to be the only independent risk factor for failing to respond to ribavirin and "low-dose" corticosteroid therapy. This is perhaps not surprising, as a high presenting LDH level has been identified as a poor prognostic indicator in this cohort, and predicted the need for ICU admission and death independently of advanced age and a high presenting neutrophil count.[8] A high LDH level on presentation may thus indicate a more complicated disease course with significant lung inflammation, necessitating more aggressive immunomodulatory therapy.

As shown by the treatment outcome of our cohort, SARS is a serious infection with a formidable morbidity and mortality. Similar to the description by Peiris *et al.*[16] and as outlined above (see section on *"Pathogenesis of disease and general treatment principles"*), the clinical course of our SARS patients appears to follow a triphasic pattern. The majority of our patients have responded to treatment, using a combination of ribavirin and intravenous steroid, during the first and second phases of their diseases, but 15.2% of our patients progressed into the third phase, characterized by development of ARDS requiring ventilatory support. Reports from several other series have also suggested that a substantial number of cases might develop respiratory failure and ARDS, with 17% to 30% of patients requiring intensive care admission,[5,13,20] whereas the 21-day mortality was reported to be 3.6%[8] and 6.5%,[13] respectively. Despite the combination of ribavirin and "low-dose" corticosteroid, the majority of our patients continued to deteriorate during the second week of the illness. High-dose methylprednisolone was used in 107 of our patients. Among them, 88.8% recovered from the progressive lung disease, and 87.7% were discharged home. Following high-dose methylprednisolone therapy, rapid resolution of lung opacity was usually followed by improvement in hypoxemia. Most of the patients responded after receiving three doses of high-dose methylprednisolone (up to 1.5 g in total). Less than 30% of cases required additional doses. Corticosteroid has been prescribed by several groups for the treatment of SARS with a favourable outcome;[5,8,9,21,22] nevertheless, some clinicians failed to observe a clinical benefit when using smaller doses of steroids than those used in our cohort.[20] Corticosteroid has been used because CT thorax findings have demonstrated radiographic features of Bronchiolitis Obliterans Organizing Pneumonia (BOOP),[8,9,23] which is a steroid responsive condition and suggestive of an immunological phenomenon.[24] The use of high-dose methylprednisolone therapy aims to suppress the cytokine-induced lung injury (phase 2)[16,22] and potentially avoid the development of ARDS (phase 3).[25] In our experience, the use of high-dose methylprednisolone during clinical progression appears effective in the majority of our cohort, but the limitation of interpreting uncontrolled data should be noted. More importantly, data is also emerging that the use of corticosteroids may even lead to worse clinical outcomes in some SARS patients [PMH SARS study group, personal communication].

The use of high dose corticosteroid therapy is not without risk or side effects. Understandably, there are concerns about using corticosteroids in treating an infectious disease.[26] In our cohort, hyperglycemia was detected in 21.5% and hypokalemia in 15% of patients while they were on steroid therapy. Two patients developed transient confusion, delusion and anxiety shortly after initiation of steroid therapy. Nosocomial infection was diagnosed in 46% of patients admitted to the intensive care unit, all of which received high dose corticosteroid therapy. Infections included pneumonia in 10 patients; predominantly caused by methicillin-resistant *S. aureus* (MRSA), bacteremia with no clearly identified site in 5 patients (MRSA in 3 patients); and urinary tract infections in two patients. The selective pressure from the antibiotics given may well explain the predominance of MRSA infection in this cohort.

The use of ribavirin in SARS is still very controversial. Ribavirin, a broad-spectrum antiviral agent previously shown to be efficacious against both RNA and DNA viruses, has been used for the treatment of SARS.[5,8,10,13,16] Previous studies have shown that in acute viral respiratory infections, large amounts of early-response cytokines such as IFN, TNF, IL–1 and IL–6 are produced. These cytokines mediate antiviral activities but at the same time may contribute to tissue injury.[27,28] Ribavirin can inhibit viral-induced macrophage production of proinflammatory cytokines and Th2 cytokines in a mouse model,[29] and thus can potentially act as an immunomodulator in addition to its antiviral effects. Nevertheless, ribavirin has been reported to have no significant *in vitro* activity against SARS-CoV. [Ref. 30, NIH communication]. In the retrospective series from Toronto, there was even a trend towards a worse outcome in those who had received ribavirin.[13] The use of high dose ribavirin can be associated with significant toxicity, including hemolysis and elevated transaminases. In our experience, after 2 weeks of ribavirin, over half of the patients developed a drop in hemoglobin level of more than $2\,g/dL$ from baseline, whereas over a third experienced a drop of more than $3\,g/dL$. Ribavirin is also teratogenic in animal models, further raising the concern whether it should be used in patients with SARS. In Canada, health officials decided on May 1 that the Special Access Programme (parenteral ribavirin is not approved for sale in Canada) will no longer provide routine access to ribavirin for the treatment of SARS [Health Canada]. Until more data from randomized controlled trials are available, physicians currently treating patients with ribavirin are strongly advised to critically re-examine the risk/benefit for each patient before continuing with the treatment.

The current recommendation from HA regarding empirical treatment of SARS is shown in Table 2. An example of an empirical treatment protocol for SARS has been published by a group of investigators in Hong Kong[21] (Table 3).

3. New treatment directions in SARS

Clearly, despite treatment with ribavirin and high dose corticosteroid therapy, up to 15%–30% of patients will not respond to therapy. These patients are at risk of developing ARDS and respiratory failure, often requiring ventilatory support in ICU. Novel treatment options and salvage therapies are urgently needed for the management of SARS patients.

In vitro testing performed recently at the USAMRIID has identified some agents with possible activity against SARS-CoV. These include alpha and beta interferons, rimantadine, and some cysteine proteinase

Table 2 Empirical Treatment of SARS*

Drug	Administration
Ribavirin	8 mg/kg every 8 hours intravenously or 1.2 g every 12 hours orally, with an oral loading dose of 4 g for those with normal renal function tests. Administer for 7–14 days depending on the response and the time of tailing off of corticosteroids.
Hydrocortisone	2 mg/kg every six hours or 4 mg/kg every 8 hours intravenously. Tail off over one week when there is clear clinical improvement. For severe and rapidly deteriorating cases, give methylprednisolone 10 mg/kg every 24 hours intravenously for two days, and then continue with hydrocortisone as above.
Antibacterial drugs	Coverage for typical and atypical agents for 7–14 days using drugs such as levofloxacin and macrolides.

Patients should be given anti-ulcer prophylaxis and monitored for hemoglobin concentration, reticulocyte count, and blood glucose and potassium concentrations. The efficacy of this regimen requires careful assessment.

* as suggested by the Hospital Authority, Hong Kong.

inhibitors [NIH communication]. Ribavirin was found to be inactive against the virus. There is currently much interest in the use of herbal medicine against SARS. Glycyrrhizin, an active component of liquorice roots, for instance, has been recently shown to be active *in vitro* against SARS-CoV.[31] A recent study by the same group of investigators also suggested that certain recombinant interferons, in particular interferon, may be active *in vitro* against SARS-CoV, and could thus be useful alone or in combination with other antiviral drugs for the treatment of SARS.[32]

Lopinavir-ritonavir (Kaletra™), a protease inhibitor widely used for treatment of HIV infection, has been shown recently to have *in vitro* activity against SARS-CoV. In a recently conducted retrospective case-control analysis in Hong Kong, the combined use of ribavirin and Kaletra (either as initial therapy, early rescue at the time of administration of pulsed steroids, or late rescue therapy after intubation) was associated with significantly better patient outcomes, in terms of reduced need for intubation and 30-days mortality.[33] Randomized controlled trials will be needed in future to clarify the role of Kaletra and other protease inhibitors in the management of SARS.

Table 3 Standard Treatment Protocol for SARS (Suspected and Probable) in Adult Patients*

(1) Antibacterial treatment
  - Start levofloxacin 500 mg once daily intravenously or orally
  - Or clarithromycin 500 mg twice daily orally plus amoxicillin and clavulanic acid 375 mg three times daily orally if patient <18 years, pregnant, or suspected to have tuberculosis

(2) Ribavirin and methylprednisolone
Add combination treatment with ribavirin and methylprednisolone when:
  - Extensive or bilateral chest radiographic involvement
  - Or persistent chest radiographic involvement and persistent high fever for 2 days
  - Or clinical, chest radiographic, or laboratory findings suggestive of worsening
  - Or oxygen saturation <95% in room air

Standard corticosteroid regimen for 21 days
  - Methylprednisolone 1 mg/kg every 8 h (3 mg/kg daily) intravenously for 5 days
  - Then methylprednisolone 1 mg/kg every 12 h (2 mg/kg daily) intravenously for 5 days
  - Then prednisolone 0.5 mg/kg twice daily (1 mg/kg daily) orally for 5 days
  - Then prednisolone 0.5 mg/kg daily orally for 3 days
  - Then prednisolone 0.25 mg/kg daily orally for 3 days
  - Then off

Ribavirin regimen for 10–14 days
  - Ribavirin 400 mg every 8 h (1200 mg daily) intravenously for at least 3 days (or until condition becomes stable)
  - Then ribavirin 1200 mg twice daily (2400 mg daily) orally

(3) Pulsed methylprednisolone
  - Give pulsed methylprednisolone if clinical condition, chest radiograph, or oxygen saturation worsens (at least two of these), and lymphopenia persists
  - Give as methylprednisolone 500 mg twice daily intravenously for 2 days, then back to standard corticosteroid regimen

(4) Ventilation
  - Consider non-invasive ventilation or mechanical ventilation if oxygen saturation <96% while on >6 L per min oxygen or if patient complains of increasing shortness of breath

Source: So *et al.*

Other agents that have been tried in SARS patients include immunomodulators such as intravenous immunoglobulin and Pentaglobin (IgM enriched immunoglobulins). It has been postulated that these compounds may act via different mechanisms in the modulation of the systemic sepsis response, including neutralizing endotoxins and exotoxins, and scavenging active complement components and lipopolysaccharides. Intravenous immunoglobulins have been used prophylactically in high-risk patients after cardiac surgery and have resulted in an improvement in infectious mortality and a reduction in mortality rate.[34] However, consistent reductions in mortality could not be demonstrated in placebo-controlled trials performed in sepsis or septic shock. These compounds have been used in SARS patient who have failed conventional therapy (e.g. IVIG 0.4 gm/kg for 5 days, or pentaglobin 300 ml IV over 12 h for 3 days). Their efficacy and safety, as well as other novel treatment strategies in SARS patients, remain to be determined, and no formal recommendations could be given for their use at this stage.

CONCLUSION

This chapter provides an overview of the current treatment strategies for SARS. The use of ribavirin is associated with significant side effects, and the lack of *in vitro* antiviral activity of ribavirin against coronavirus has rendered its role doubtful in the treatment of SARS. The use of high-dose methylprednisolone during clinical progression, with the rationale to prevent immunopathological lung injury, appears effective in our limited experience, but again caution is required before further generalization or recommendations could be made based on these findings. Randomized controlled studies will be required to evaluate the efficacy and best timing for high-dose methylprednisolone therapy, as well as the utility of novel antiviral agents. For those with progressive disease, novel immunomodulatory agents could be considered as salvage therapy. The availability of the genome sequence of the SARS coronavirus will hopefully facilitate efforts to develop new and rapid diagnostic tests, antiviral agents and vaccines in the long run.

REFERENCES

1. Kuiken T, Fouchier RAM, Schutten M, *et al*. Newly discovered coronavirus as the primary cause of severe acute respiratory syndrome. *Lancet* 2003;**362**(9380):263–70.

2. Rota PA, Oberste MS, Monroe SS, *et al*. Characterization of a novel coronavirus associated with severe acute respiratory syndrome. *Science*. 2003;**300**(5624):1394–9. Epub 2003 May 01.

3. Marra MA, Jones SJ, Astell CR, *et al*. The Genome sequence of the SARS-associated coronavirus. *Science*. 2003;**300**(5624):1399–404. Epub 2003 May 01.

4. Anand K, Ziebuhr J, Wadhwani P, *et al*. Coronavirus main proteinase (3CLpro) structure: Basis for design of anti-SARS drugs. *Science* 2003;**300**(5626):1763–7. Epub 2003 May 13.

5. Peiris JS, Lai ST, Poon LL, *et al*. Coronavirus as a possible cause of severe acute respiratory syndrome. *Lancet* 2003;**361**(9366):1319–25.

6. Ksiazek TG, Erdman D, Goldsmith CS, *et al*. A novel coronavirus associated with severe acute respiratory syndrome. *N Engl J Med* 2003;**348**(20):1953–66. Epub 2003 Apr 10.

7. Drosten C, Gunther S, Preiser W, *et al*. Identification of a novel coronavirus in patients with severe acute respiratory syndrome. *N Engl J Med* 2003;**348**:1967–76.

8. Lee N, Hui D, Wu A, *et al*. A major outbreak of severe acute respiratory syndrome in Hong Kong. *N Engl J Med* 2003;**348**(20):1986–94. Epub 2003 Apr 07.

9. Tsang KW, Ho PL, Ooi GC, *et al*. A cluster of cases of severe acute respiratory syndrome in Hong Kong. *N Engl J Med* 2003;**348**(20):1977–85. Epub 2003 Mar 31.

10. Poutanen SM, Low DE, Henry B, *et al*. Identification of severe acute respiratory syndrome in Canada. *N Engl J Med* 2003;**348**(20): 1995–2005. Epub 2003 Mar 31.

11. Hon KL, Leung CW, Cheng WT, *et al*. Clinical presentations and outcome of severe acute respiratory syndrome in children. *Lancet* 2003;**361**(9370):1701–3.

12. Rickerts V, Wolf T, Rottmann C, *et al*. Clinical presentation and management of the severe acute respiratory syndrome (SARS). *Dtsch Med Wochenschr* 2003;**128**(20):1109–14.

13. Booth CM, Matukas LM, Tomlinson GA, *et al*. Clinical features and short-term outcomes of 144 patients with SARS in the greater Toronto area. *JAMA* 2003;**289**(21):2801–9. Epub 2003 May 06.

14. The Acute Respiratory Distress Syndrome Network. Ventilation with lower tidal volumes as compared with traditional tidal volumes for acute lung injury and the acute respiratory distress syndrome. *N Engl J Med* 2000;**342**:1301–8.

15. Joseph JY Sung. Severe acute respiratory syndrome: What do we know about this disease? *HK Med Diary* 2003;**8**:15–6.

16. Peiris JS, Chu CM, Cheng VC, *et al.* Clinical progression and viral load in a community outbreak of coronavirus-associated SARS pneumonia: A prospective study. *Lancet.* 2003;**361**(9371):1767–72.

17. Nicholls JM, Poon LL, Lee KC, *et al.* Lung pathology of fatal severe acute respiratory syndrome. *Lancet* 2003;**361**:1773–8.

18. Guidelines for the management of adults with community-acquired pneumonia: Diagnosis, assessment of severity, antimicrobial therapy, and prevention. *Am J Respir Crit Care Med* 2001;**163**:1730–54.

19. The Acute Respiratory Distress Syndrome Network. Ventilation with lower tidal volumes as compared with traditional tidal volumes for acute lung injury and the acute respiratory distress syndrome. *N Engl J Med* 2000;**342**:1301–8.

20. Hsu LY, Lee CC, Green JA, *et al.* Severe acute respiratory syndrome in Singapore: Clinical features of index patient and initial contacts. *Emerg Infect Dis* 2003;**9**:713–7.

21. So LK, Lau AC, Yam LY, *et al.* Development of a standard treatment protocol for severe acute respiratory syndrome. *Lancet* 2003;**361**: 1615–7.

22. Zhong NS, Zeng GQ. Our strategies for fighting severe acute respiratory syndrome. *Am J Respir Crit Care Med* 2003: http://ajrccm.atsjournals.org/cgi/reprint/200305-707OEv1.pdf. (Accessed May 28, 2003).

23. Wong KT, Antonio GE, Hui DS, *et al.* Thin-section CT of severe acute respiratory syndrome: Evaluation of 73 patients exposed to or with the disease. *Radiology* 2003: http://radiology.rsnajnls.org/cgi/content/full/2283030541v1. (Accessed May 12, 2003).

24. Epler GR. Bronchiolitis obliterans organizing pneumonia. *Arch Intern Med* 2001;**161**:158–64.

25. Marks JD, Marks CB, Luce JM, *et al.* Plasma tumor necrosis factor in patients with septic shock: Mortality rate, incidence of adult respiratory distress syndrome. *Am Rev Respir Dis* 1990;**141**:94–7.

26. Oba Y. The use of corticosteroids in SARS. *N Engl J Med* 2003; **348**(20):2034–5; author's reply, 2034–5.

27. Cheung CY, Poon LL, Lau AS, *et al*. Induction of proinflammatory cytokines in human macrophage by influenza A (H5N1) virus: A mechanism for the unusual severity of human disease? *Lancet* 2002; **360**:1831–7.

28. Van Reeth K, Van Gucht S, Pensaret M. *In vivo* studies on cytokines involvement during acute viral respiratory infection of swine: Troublesome but rewarding. *Vet Immune Immunopath* 2002;**87**:161–8.

29. Ning Q, Brown D, Parodo J, *et al*. Ribavirin inhibits viral-induced macrophage production of TNF, IL-1, the procoagulant fg12 pro-thrombinase and preserves Th1 cytokine production but inhibits Th2 cytokine response. *J Immunol* 1998;**160**:3487–93.

30. Cyranoski D. Critics slam treatment for SARS as infective and perhaps dangerous. *Nature* 2003;**423**:4.

31. Cinatl J, Morgenstern B, Bauer G, *et al*. Glycyrrhizin, an active component of liquorice roots, and replication of SARS-associated coronavirus. *Lancet* 2003;**361**:2045–6.

32. Cinatl J, Morgenstern B, Bauer G, *et al*. Treatment of SARS with human interferons. *Lancet* 2003;**362**(9380):293–4.

33. Sung J. Clinical diagnosis and management of SARS. WHO Global Conference on Severe Acute Respiratory Syndrome (SARS). 17–18 June 2003. Kuala Lumpur. (Accessed online at: http://SARSreference.com/link.php?id=18.)

34. Pilz G, Kreuzer E, Kaab S, *et al*. Early sepsis treatment with immunoglobulins after cardiac surgery in score-identified high-risk patients. *Chest* 1994;**105**(1):76–82. Erratum in: *Chest* 1994;**105**(6):1924.

11

The Clinical Management of SARS

Gavin M Joynt, Charles D Gomersall

Severe acute respiratory syndrome (SARS) is a new infectious disease most likely caused by the SARS coronavirus.[1-3] The disease is readily transmissible and rapidly spread throughout the world.[4] The resulting outbreak has now been contained worldwide; however, the risk of recurrence of the outbreak remains. During the recent outbreak, a high proportion of cases, approximately 20%, required intensive care unit (ICU) admission.[5] The provision of organ support in the ICU, therefore, plays a potentially important role in reducing mortality, which has been reported to be 10% for younger patients and as high as 50% for patients above 60 years old.[6] At the time of writing, there are little published data on ICU management and outcome of SARS,[7,8] and much of the information that follows is based largely on observational data derived from our institution.

ICU ADMISSION CRITERIA AND DEMOGRAPHICS

The clinical presentation of patients with SARS has been described elsewhere.[5,9] The usual CDC case definition of clinical, epidemiologic and laboratory features for the diagnosis of SARS were present in all patients admitted to the ICU during the outbreak.[10]

SARS is a progressive disease and the average interval from the onset of symptoms to requirement for ICU admission was approximately 10 days, similar to the 8 days reported recently in Singapore and Toronto.[7,8] While fever and other systemic symptoms tended to improve during the first week, particularly in response to steroid therapy, the more important markers of clinical deterioration were manifested by progressive hypoxia and dyspnea, accompanied by the progression of pulmonary infiltrates on chest radiograph.[5] Several features present at admission are associated with the likelihood of ICU admission or death. These include older age, presence of comorbidity (particularly diabetes), bilateral infiltrates at the time of admission, elevated LDH, and higher absolute neutrophil count.[5,7,8] It has been suggested that a higher viral load may be associated with a more severe disease.[7] Close monitoring of chest radiographs and respiratory function parameters in the general wards was, therefore, important to detect ongoing deterioration in those patients who were eventually admitted to ICU.

Admission to ICU was invariably the consequence of progressive, severe respiratory failure unresponsive to the administration of moderate concentrations of inspired oxygen. In general, patients were admitted following: (1) failure to maintain an arterial oxygen saturation of at least 90% while receiving supplemental oxygen of 50%; and/or (2) demonstration of a respiratory rate greater than 35 breaths per minute.

The ICU admission rate was 20% and the average age of patients at ICU admissions (approximately 50 years, with a range of 23 to 81 years), was similar to results reported from Singapore and Toronto.[7,8] An approximately equal number of males and females have been admitted. A typical admission APACHE II score was a moderate 10–12. This was lower than the APACHE II scores of 18–19 reported recently,[7,8] and the reason for this apparent difference is unclear as a greater number of our patients (more than 90%) met the clinical criteria for ARDS: acute onset of bilateral diffuse pulmonary infiltrates on chest radiograph; an arterial oxygen tension to fractional inspired oxygen concentration (PaO_2/FiO_2) ratio of less than 200 mmHg; and the absence of left atrial hypertension.[11] The most remarkable feature of these patients was the predominance of isolated respiratory failure. The multiple organ dysfunction (MOD) score,[12] scores six organ systems on a scale of 0–4, giving a maximum score of 24 points. For patients assessed so far, the median MOD score in the first 24 h is 3, with the majority of points being derived from the respiratory system.

ICU MANAGEMENT AND PROGRESS

Medical therapy for SARS in the ICU is evolving, and there is no evidence to support the use of any specific regimen. In the ICU, medical therapy was an extension of the protocol utilized in the general ward.[5] This included the use of broad-spectrum antibiotics (to provide therapy for the usual causes of community acquired pneumonia), ribavirin and low dose corticosteroids. In addition, methylprednisolone 500 mg to 1 g daily for two to three days, was used in an attempt to dampen the inflammatory response in those patients who continue to deteriorate. Deterioration was generally manifested by worsening hypoxia, respiratory distress, and worsening opacities on chest radiograph. High-dose methylprednisolone was occasionally repeated in the most severe cases, to a total dosage of 5 g. Some of these cases also received convalescent plasma donated by patients who had recovered from SARS and/or IgM enriched immunoglobulin. Broad-spectrum antibiotics (cefepime, carbapenem, or fluoroquinolone) were administered at the time of institution of high dose pulse methyl-prednisolone therapy, but were withdrawn in the absence of obvious clini-cal sepsis in the first 3 to 5 days following high-dose methylprednisolone therapy. Suspected ICU nosocomial infection was treated early with empirical board spectrum antibiotics (cefepime, carbapenem, or fluoro-quinolone plus an aminoglycoside) and if necessary, vancomycin and anti-fungal agents. The antibiotic regimen was modified according to the results of bacterial culture of sputum, tracheal aspirate and blood.

OXYGENATION AND VENTILATORY SUPPORT

Supportive management in the ICU focused on oxygen supplementation and, when absolutely necessary, mechanical ventilation. Initially, oxygen supplementation was provided using nasal cannulae, and where necessary Hudson type masks. Patients requiring very high inspired oxygen concen-trations were provided with non-rebreathing masks fitted with a reservoir. The use of entrainment or Venturi-type masks was avoided as the high gas flows generated might encourage dispersal of contaminated droplets dur-ing coughing or sneezing. Noninvasive positive pressure ventilation was also avoided because of the risk of viral transmission potentially resulting from mask leakage and high gas-flow compensation, possibly causing wide dispersion of contaminated aerosol. Later in the course of the epi-demic, an oxygen delivery device was developed that allowed both the delivery of high flow oxygen to the patient and filtration of expired gases by a high quality bacterial and viral humidifier/filter (Fig. 1).

The decision to initiate intubation and mechanical ventilation was a clinical one. The criteria for intubation and positive pressure ventilation were: (1) persistent failure to achieve arterial oxygen saturation of 90% while receiving 100% oxygen via a non-rebreathing mask; and/or (2) onset of respiratory muscle fatigue as evidenced by an increase in arterial carbon dioxide tension ($PaCO_2$), sweating, tachycardia and/or a subjective feeling of exhaustion. While these indications lead to intubation relatively later than might be usually expected, mechanical ventilation was required in 50–60% of the patients admitted to the ICU. Leaving the decision to institute intubation and ventilation late might be potentially

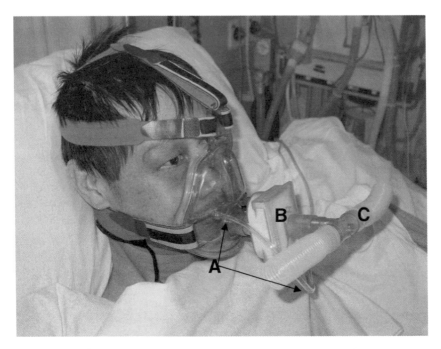

Fig. 1 Modified mask arrangement to enable high inspired oxygen concentrations to be provided to the patient while protecting the environment from excess viral contamination. Picture courtesy of originator, Dr. CD Gomersall. The tightly fitting mask is a standard mask used for non-invasive ventilation. Note A, the oxygen supply tubing (oxygen is supplied at 15 L/min); B, the high quality humidifier and bacterial/viral filter; and C, the T-piece reservoir arrangement. Close supervision of patients is required in ICU.

dangerous if certain precautions are not taken. Particular attention was paid to the pre-emptive assessment of the likely difficulty of intubation of individual patients. All the patients were closely monitored by experienced nurses on a one-to-one basis, and all necessary intubation and personal protective equipment was readily available at the bedside of the more severe patients. Availability of experienced doctors with airway expertise was ensured at all times.

Usually, mechanical ventilation with synchronized intermittent mandatory ventilation (SIMV), or pressure control ventilation, was instituted. Positive end expiratory pressure (PEEP) and inspired oxygen concentration was titrated to achieve an arterial saturation of 90–95%. The aim of limiting barotrauma and volutrauma as much as possible was pursued by instituting low-pressure, low-volume ventilation, based on the principles of the ARDS-net study. Tidal volume was maintained at 6–8 ml/kg estimated body weight, and plateau pressure was limited at 30 cm H_2O or less. $PaCO_2$ was allowed to rise if necessary, provided the pH was greater than 7.15.[13] A small number of patients unable to meet the above parameters were ventilated in a prone position.

CIRCULATORY SUPPORT AND FLUID MANAGEMENT

Fluid intake and losses were strictly controlled with the aim of maintaining an intake/output balance of approximately nil. Vasopressors at small to moderate doses were used to maintain adequate blood pressure in preference to the use of bolus fluid infusion. Patients were otherwise managed according to standard ICU organ support protocols.

NOSOCOMIAL INFECTION

Nosocomial infection rates appeared higher than baseline rates in the ICU, although the data to confirm this has not yet been formally analyzed. Ventilator associated pneumonia occurred in approximately 20% of cases; urinary tract infection in 5% of cases; catheter related infections in 5% of cases; and primary bacteremia in about 12% of cases. Duration of stay in ICU was longer than usual and may contribute to the apparently high infection rates. Prior to the outbreak, *Pseudomonas aeruginosa* had been a commonly cultured nosocomial organism, but was rarely seen after the outbreak. Common organisms cultured during the outbreak included *Staphylococcus aureus*, *Stenotrophomonas maltophilia* and *Candida albicans*. The high incidence of nosocomial infection may have been caused by the use of high-dose steroid therapy. It could also be a consequence of the immunosuppressive effects of the disease itself.

OUTCOME AND RECOMMENDATIONS

Almost all the patients admitted to the ICU for SARS met the criteria for acute respiratory distress syndrome (ARDS) during the ICU stay. The plain radiograph features of established SARS in the ICU are indistinguishable from those of ARDS. The typical features of ARDS include bilateral widespread, confluent opacification, with the lung periphery being denser or more extensively involved than the perihilar regions. Unfortunately, no CT images were available for ICU patients in the early acute stage of ARDS; however, in some of the early deaths, post-mortem histology demonstrated changes consistent with the early and organizing phase of diffuse alveolar damage. The early phase was characterized by pulmonary edema with hyaline membrane formation, suggestive of the acute stage of ARDS, while cellular fibromyxoid organizing exudates in the air spaces indicated the organizing phase that follows alveolar damage.[5] Multinucleated pneumocytes are common and SARS is also associated with epithelial-cell proliferation and an increase in macrophages in the alveoli and the interstitium of the lung.[14]

The pneumothorax rate in ventilated patients was approximately 20%. Barotrauma was reported in 20% of ventilator cases in Singapore and 34% in Toronto.[7,8] This is substantially higher than that reported previously in ventilated patients with ARDS.[15,16] This occurred despite relatively late mechanical ventilation and close attention to the limitation of excess pressure and volume during mechanical ventilation. At present there is no obvious explanation for this observation, but the relatively high rate of pneumothorax in mechanically ventilated cases, coupled with the observation of barotrauma in a non-ventilated case, suggests that care needs to be taken to avoid circumstances that might exacerbate the risk of barotrauma. Avoiding mechanical ventilation as much as possible and if required, utilizing low-volume, low-pressure ventilation would seem prudent. Daily chest radiographs may facilitate the early detection of barotrauma and avoid progression to complications, such as tension pneumothorax.

Based on the survival rate in the first 50 patients who were admitted to our ICU, the mortality rate from SARS in ICU is expected to be about

30%. This compares with 37% 28-day mortality in Singapore and 34% in Toronto.[7,8] The ultimate cause of death was usually the result of oxygenation failure, complications of pre-existing comorbid disease, or organ failure as a consequence of nosocomial sepsis.

It is difficult to objectively assess whether the specific medical regimen of broad spectrum antibiotics, followed by ribavirin, corticosteroid and intermittent high-dose corticosteroid therapy, had a positive effect on patient outcome. No controlled study was attempted in view of the sudden, severe and unexpected nature of the outbreak. Anecdotally, the effect of high-dose methylprednisolone was impressive in reducing inspired oxygen requirements and rapidly reversing radiographic opacities in a number of patients. An example of this type of response is show in Fig. 2. A more detailed description of the response to medical therapy used in this institution can be found in the chapter on medical management. It should be noted that ribavirin therapy was discontinued in Singapore, in view of its perceived lack of efficacy,[7] and that high-dose pulse methylprednisolone was rarely used in the Toronto outbreak.[8] Outcome differences between the three centers appear similar.

The median maximal MOD score during the ICU stay in the cohort of patients assessed so far was 5 (out of a possible 24 — see earlier

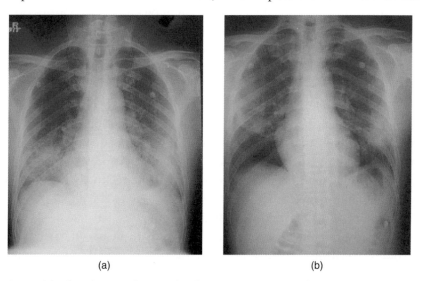

(a)   (b)

Fig. 2 (a) The chest radiograph of this male patient demonstrates severe bilateral pulmonary infiltrates. (b) A chest radiograph 24 hours following 1g high-dose methylprednisolone therapy. The patients oxygen requirement was also markedly reduced.

explanation), with the majority of the score being made up of the respiratory component, again indicating the relative lack of organ failure outside the respiratory system. The average length of stay in the ICU for all patients was approximately 10 days, similar to that reported from Toronto.[8] Those patients who required mechanical ventilation, however, remained in the ICU for an average of two weeks. A large number of mechanically ventilated patients, therefore, progressed beyond the acute stage and into the chronic stages of ARDS.[17] In general, the CT features of late stage ARDS caused by SARS (Fig. 3) were similar to those seen in late stage ARDS from other causes.[18,19] Interestingly, the severe CT changes of late stage ARDS were seen even in patients not mechanically ventilated.

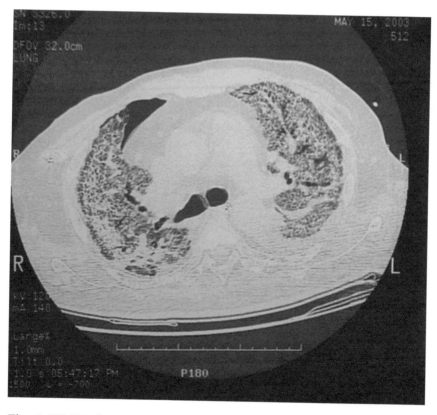

Fig. 3 HRCT of a 56-year-old man in the chronic phase of ARDS from SARS. This patient was receiving high concentrations of oxygen and mechanical ventilation. Multiple small cysts are present. There is architectural distortion, volume loss, bronchiectasis, parenchymal bands and irregularly thickened interlobular septae. Extrapleural gas is visible.

At this stage, the outcome of the patients with late stage ARDS from SARS is unknown; however, one patient who was ventilated for over 100 days, has been successfully weaned from the ventilator and discharged to the ward in stable condition. Notable complications from prolonged ventilation and the use of deep sedation and paralysis necessary to allow the end points of low-pressure, low-volume ventilation to be met, were neuromuscular weakness and severe muscle wasting. The use of high-dose methylprednisolone is likely to have contributed to the neuromuscular weakness observed. Prolonged weaning and the need for active mobilization and rehabilitation were frequently necessary for this group of patients.

INFECTION CONTROL IN THE ICU

The objectives of infection control in the ICU are to prevent transmission of SARS from patients to visitors, staff or other patients in the ICU. This can be achieved by introducing a variety of measures that include patient isolation, environmental protection and personal protection. SARS is readily transmissible and the virus has been detected in blood, respiratory secretions, feces, urine and various tissue specimens. High viral RNA concentrations have been detected in respiratory secretions and feces.[2] Spread probably occurs most frequently via droplets and aerosols, which may be enhanced by the use of nebulizers or similar devices.[20] Spread has also been linked to contaminated sewage systems.[21] The virus is stable on surfaces for days after shedding and so contact with infected surfaces could also be a possible source of contamination.

Details of infection control procedures used in the ICU of the Prince of Wales Hospital can be obtained online,[22] but some of the most important issues and recommendations, based on our observations, are summarized here.

If possible, patients should be isolated in single rooms. Air pressure in isolation rooms should be negative compared with pressure in the surrounding areas. Air changes should be adequate and at least 6–12 air changes per hour are recommended. There should also be appropriate discharge of air outdoors or monitored high-efficiency filtration of isolation room air before the air is re-circulated. Although these are high-grade recommendations,[23] we believe they can be justified in the context of our experience of SARS. If isolation rooms are not available, it appears reasonable to isolate the patients in a unit so that they would not be in contact with other patients. Access to isolation areas must be strictly controlled. The ICU itself should only be accessible to staff directly involved in patient care to prevent unnecessary exposure. Visitors should not be allowed.

Personal protective equipment such as N95 or higher grade mask respirators, caps, tight fitting goggles or full face shields, shoe covers, disposable water-resistant gowns and gloves should be readily available and all staff, including visiting staff such as physiotherapists and radiographers should undergo proper training in the use of personal protective equipment. Initial, formal mask "fit-test" with a commercially available kit should be performed to ensure proper mask size and fit for each individual expected to enter the ICU environment. Close supervision of activities in a designated "gown-up" and separated "gown-down" areas should be provided. When exiting the ICU, the "gown-down" area should also be regulated and monitored. Inanimate objects must either be placed in a protective covering or be properly cleansed when a staff leaves a high-risk area.

Infection control training is essential and should cover not only procedural requirements, but also provide information relating to the SARS coronavirus and possible modes of transmission, to ensure informed adherence to infection control rules. Infection control behavior in the ICU must be regularly audited and repeatedly enforced. Regular hand cleansing and glove changing between patient contacts is essential but commonly forgotten or avoided as it is time consuming and inconvenient. All clinical areas and equipment should be disinfected regularly and thoroughly with chlorine or hypochlorite solutions.[24]

Avoidance of, or at a minimum, extra care needs to be taken if it is necessary to come into contact with patients undergoing procedures that may enhance the dissemination of contaminated aerosols. This includes the use of entrainment oxygen devices, nebulizers, noninvasive ventilation, intubation and bronchoscopic procedures. It has been suggested that intubation, particularly difficult intubation, might be associated with a higher risk of spread.[8] During intubation and resuscitation, all staff are required to wear hoods, in addition to other personal protective equipment (Fig. 4). After a high risk procedure, staff are encouraged to change all personal protective equipment, take a shower and put on fresh clothing as soon as possible.

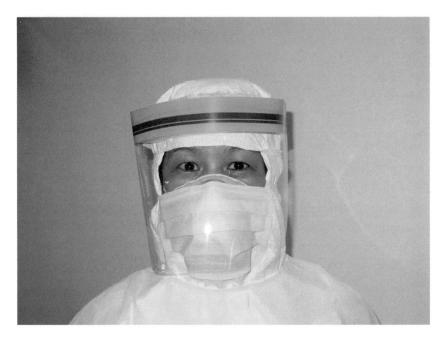

Fig. 4 A protective hood in situ. Note the N95 respirator worn under the hood, which is only provided with a protective surgical mask.

High quality bacterial and viral filters are used to minimize environmental contamination in patients requiring mechanical ventilation. We utilize hydrophobic filters with greater than 99.99999% filtration capacity. Heat and moisture exchanging filters are used at the endotracheal tube ventilator circuit interface and an additional filter is placed at the ventilator expiratory port. Filters should also be used when manual ventilation with a bag valve resuscitator is needed. Closed suction systems for tracheal suction are utilized.

Infection control precautions must be maintained during transport of patients outside the ICU, and all ICU transport and receiving radiology suite staff should be attired in full personal protective clothing and equipment. Staff must be warned to take special precautions in areas where close personal contact may occur outside the ICU. Special eating cubicles were constructed in the ICU common room to facilitate safe eating (Fig. 5). Instructions on tea room and social behavior, such as bathroom hygiene, maintaining adequate distance between staff while eating, non-sharing of food and utensils, and instruction to wear a mask whenever possible were

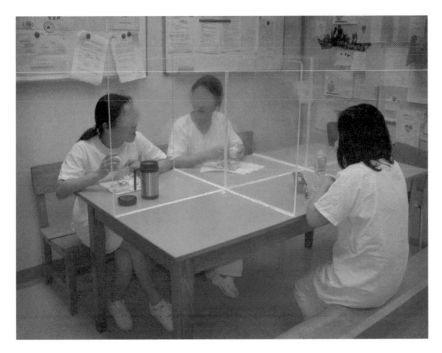

Fig. 5 A cubicle arrangement in the ICU tea room. Individual eating areas are washed with hypochlorite solution before and after use.

issued.[25] A similar set of guidelines on simple precautions to take when returning home to families was also distributed.

Five of approximately 280 staff regularly exposed to the ICU during the outbreak contracted SARS. There were no fatalities. Four of the five contracted the disease within a few weeks of the start of the outbreak. No family members were known to have been infected by ICU staff.

CONCLUSIONS AND FUTURE IMPLICATIONS

SARS is a serious infectious disease that causes predominantly severe respiratory failure, with little other organ failure. Admission rates to ICU are high and the morbidity and mortality are significant. The clinical picture in ICU resembles ARDS; however, there appears to be a high incidence of barotrauma, particularly amongst those patients requiring mechanical ventilation. Nosocomial infection rates appear high, and may be disease- or therapy related. SARS and possibly other similar new diseases in the future have important implications for ICU provision. Certainly in high-risk areas, it will become necessary to ensure that future infection control practice continues to protect staff from possible new cases. This implies continued vigilance and the continued maintenance of some or all of the above measures, but ultimately the risk of infection will have to be balanced by measures that are practical and sustainable. Design of hospitals and ICUs in particular, will have to account for the requirements of effective isolation. Contingency for the sudden increase in requirements for ICU services, such as occurred in SARS, will have to be developed. In summary, SARS has highlighted the need for serious reconsideration of strategic ICU planning in the future.

REFERENCES

1. Peiris JS, Lai ST, Poon LL, *et al.* Coronavirus as a possible cause of severe acute respiratory syndrome. *Lancet* 2003;**361**:1319–25.

2. Drosten C, Gunther S, Preiser W, *et al.* Identification of a novel coronavirus in patients with severe acute respiratory syndrome. *N Engl J Med* 2003;**348**:1967–76.

3. Fouchier RA, Kuiken T, Schutten M, *et al.* Aetiology: Koch's postulates fulfilled for SARS virus. *Nature* 2003;**423**:240.

4. Centers for Disease Control and Prevention. CDC update: Outbreak of severe acute respiratory syndrome-worldwide, 2003. *MMWR* 2003; **52**:241–8.

5. Lee N, Hui D, Wu A, *et al.* A major outbreak of severe acute respiratory syndrome in Hong Kong. *N Engl J Med* 2003;**348**:1986–94.

6. Donnelly CA, Ghani AC, Leung GM, *et al.* Epidemiological determinants of spread of causal agent of severe acute respiratory syndrome. *Lancet* 2003;**361**:1761–6.

7. Lew TWK, Kwek T-K, Tai D, *et al.* Acute respiratory distress syndrome in critically ill patients with severe acute respiratory syndrome. *JAMA* 2003;**290**:374–80.

8. Fowler RA, Lapinsky SE, Hallett D, *et al.* Critically ill patients with severe acute respiratory syndrome. *JAMA* 2003;**290**:367–73.

9. Booth CM, Matukas LM, Tomlinson GA, *et al.* Clinical features and short-term outcomes of 144 patients with SARS in the greater Toronto area. *JAMA* 2003;**289**:2801–9.

10. Centers for Disease Control and Prevention. Updated interim US case definition for severe acute respiratory syndrome (SARS)-update, April 30, 2003: http://www.cdc.gov/ncidod/sars/casedefinition.htm (accessed May 10, 2003).

11. Bernard GR, Artigas A, Brigham KL, *et al.* The American-European Consensus Conference on ARDS. Definitions, mechanisms, relevant outcomes, and clinical trial coordination. *Am J Respir Crit Care Med* 1994;**149**(3 Pt 1):818–24.

12. Marshall JC, Cook DJ, Christou NV, *et al.* Multiple organ dysfunction score: A reliable descriptor of a complex clinical outcome. *Crit Care Med* 1995;**23**(10):1638–52.

13. Ventilation with lower tidal volume as compared with traditional tidal volumes for acute lung injury and the acute respiratory distress syndrome: The acute respiratory distress syndrome network. *New Engl J Med* 2000;**342**:1301–08.

14. Nicholls JM, Poon LL, Lee KC, *et al.* Lung pathology of fatal severe acute respiratory syndrome. *Lancet* 2003;**361**:1773–8.

15. Weg JG, Anzueto A, Balk RA, *et al.* The relations of pneumothorax and other air leaks to mortality in the acute respiratory distress syndrome. *N Engl J Med* 1998;**338**:341–6.

16. Stewart TE, Meade MO, Cook DJ, *et al.* Evaluation of a ventilation strategy to prevent barotrauma in patients at high risk for acute respiratory distress syndrome. *N Engl J Med* 1998;**338**:355–61.

17. Gattinoni L, Bombino M, Pelosi P, *et al.* Lung structure and function in different stages of severe adult respiratory distress syndrome. *JAMA* 1994;**271**:1772–9.

18. Gattinoni L, Caironi P, Pelosi P, Goodman LR. What has computed tomography taught us about the acute respiratory distress syndrome? *Am J Respir Crit Care Med* 2001;**164**:1701–11.

19. Rouby J, Puybasset L, Nieszkowska A. Acute respiratory distress syndrome: Lessons from computed tomography of the whole lung. *Crit Care Med* 2003;**31**(4) (Suppl.) S285–95.

20. Tomlinson B, Cockram C. SARS: Experience at Prince of Wales Hospital, Hong Kong. *Lancet* 2003;**361**:1486–87.

21. Hong Kong Department of Health Report. Main findings of an investigation into the outbreak of severe acute respiratory syndrome

at Amoy Gardens. http://www.info.gov.hk/dh/ap.htm (accessed April 19, 2003).

22. Joynt GM, Gomersall CD. Severe acute respiratory syndrome (SARS). http://www.aic.cuhk.edu.hk/web8/sudden_acute_respiratory_ syndrom.htm.

23. Garner JS, Hospital Infection Control Practices Advisory Commitee. Guideline for isolation precautions in hospitals. *Infect Control Hosp Epidemiol* 1996;**17**:53–80, and *Am J Infect Control* 1996;**24**:24–52.

24. Hospital infection control guidance for severe acute respiratory syndrome (SARS) http://www.who.int/csr/sars/infectioncontrol/en. (accessed April 11, 2003).

25. Li TS, Buckley TA, Yap FH, Sung JJ, Joynt GM. Severe acute respiratory syndrome (SARS): Infection control. *Lancet* 2003;**361**:1386.

12

Severe Acute Respiratory Syndrome in Elderly Patients

Timothy Kwok

EPIDEMIOLOGY

According to the Hospital Authority database of 1315 confirmed cases of SARS in Hong Kong in 2003, 14% of the victims were people aged 65 years or above. Forty four percent of them contracted the disease during hospital stay, indicating that cross infection in the hospital setting was a very important cause of SARS in older people. Because of this, a lot of older people with SARS were frail and had significant comorbidity. Overall, 16% of the older SARS patients were old-age home residents. Fifty-five percent of these old-age home residents contracted the virus in hospitals, suggesting that there were also some cross infections of SARS in the old-age home setting.

CLINICAL FEATURES

The clinical features of SARS in older people were slightly different from those of younger people. Based on the above Hospital Authority database of confirmed cases of SARS patients, the symptomatology of older and

159

Table 1 Comparison of Presenting Symptoms of SARS in 184 Older and 1131 Young People with Confirmed SARS in Hong Kong *

Symptom	Old (%)	Young (%)	p Value
Fever	76	90	0.00
Cough	34	42	0.04
Malaise	32	56	0.00
Chill	27	62	0.00
Sputum	24	20	0.17
Breathless	22	9	0.00
Diarrhoea	11	16	0.03
Vomiting	7	11	0.07

*Subjects aged 65 years or older were defined as older people.

younger people was compared in Table 1. Older patients were less likely to report specific symptoms. On the other hand, atypical symptoms were not uncommon — decreased general condition (17%), poor feeding (10%), delirium (3%) and fall (1%). Because many older patients contracted SARS during hospital stay (44%) and many older SARS patients were old-age home residents (16%), hospital stay in the preceding two weeks and old-age home residence were important risk factors of SARS in older people.

As in other infections in older people, fever was less pronounced and might be absent. This problem was compounded by the common use of axillary temperature in hospitals, which was more subject to measurement error in thin and uncooperative patients. Interestingly, a rise in pulse rate in the absence of fever was noted in 18% of the older SARS patients. The official definition of clinical SARS requires a body temperature of 38°C or more. This will lead to late or missed diagnosis in older people. A temperature rise of more than 1°C above the baseline may be more sensitive.

The incubation period in older people may be longer than the maximum of ten days in younger people. An incubation period as long as three weeks has been reported. However, there are problems in determining the incubation period in older people because the symptoms and fever can easily be missed, for example, the onset of fever is frequently taken as the onset of the disease. But the fever pattern has been described as biphasic. If the first phase of fever presumably from viremia is somehow missed, late presentation with the second phase of fever may lead to an impression of a long incubation period. Furthermore the older people in hospital and old age home may have exposure to SARS at different time points, thus making the timing of exposure uncertain.

The mortality rate of SARS in older people was very high, ranging from 50–75%. Late presentation and comorbidities were likely to be contributory. Moreover, they were likely to suffer from side effects of medical treatment used for SARS, e.g. Ribavirin and steroids. The risk and benefit ratio of any treatment for SARS in older people is therefore more finely balanced.

Older people are a heterogeneous group. The clinical features of fit older people were similar to those of younger people. But the diagnosis of SARS was more problematic in the frail older people. Firstly, as previously mentioned, they were unlikely to report symptoms because of cognitive impairment, dysphasia or dsyarthria. Secondly, there are a variety of conditions e.g. aspiration pneumonia associated with dysphagia, tuberculosis, chronic lung diseases, which can give rise to recurrent fever and thus confuse the clinical picture. Thirdly, lymphopenia which was a commonly used diagnostic feature of SARS is common among geriatric patients and is related to malnutrition and frailty. Fourthly, the presentations of SARS may be atypical, e.g. falls, confusion and incontinence. A fall may result in a hip or vertebral fracture and lead to admission to an orthopedic hospital ward. Acute confusion in a demented patient may lead to admission to a psychogeriatric ward.

Because of these diagnostic difficulties and the lack of an effective early diagnostic test during the previous outbreak, many older patients were under suspicion of SARS and the detection of SARS was delayed in some cases, thus increasing the risk of cross infection in the interim period.

From the point of view of infection control, the care of the frail older people in the hospital and old-age home settings was particularly challenging. Assisting these people in the activities of daily living, e.g. feeding, bathing and transferring, involves close personal contacts. The confused patients could not comply with any infection control measures, e.g. wearing face masks, confining themselves in cohorted areas. This posed a great infection risk for their caregivers and the people around them.

OLD-AGE HOMES

Old-age home residents are generally frail and have high hospital admission rates. The chances of contracting SARS through cross infection in old-age homes were therefore significant. Overall, the prevalence of SARS among old-age home residents was more than three times that of the general population. Considering that there were more than 50,000 old-age home residents in Hong Kong, the risk of the spread of SARS in this setting was a major worry.

The Hospital Authority and the Department of Health took the following steps to prevent the spread of SARS in old-age homes:

1. Infection control measures in all old-age homes, e.g. hand washing, wearing of face mask, daily temperature measurement were stepped up, with the support and encouragement from the community geriatric team and the Department of Health.
2. All residents discharged from hospitals were kept under close surveillance in a cohorted area for a minimum of ten days.
3. All residents in close or social contact with SARS patients in hospitals were monitored for ten days in the hospitals before they were discharged.
4. All old-age home residents were screened by geriatricians before they were discharged from hospitals.
5. A daily territory-wise updated database of confirmed or suspected SARS cases in old-age homes was communicated to geriatric teams.

While it was important to send SARS patients to hospitals for appropriate medical management and to prevent cross infection in old-age homes, it was equally important to avoid inappropriate hospital admissions which put the older residents at risk of contracting SARS. Afterall, old-age home residents are more likely to have fever not related to SARS, because of concomitant diseases. Therefore, the medical support for old-age homes was stepped up through enhanced outreach activities by geriatric nurses and geriatricians. Private practitioners were also employed to provide frequent on site primary healthcare support and to ensure compliance with infection control measures.

PSYCHOLOGICAL CONSEQUENCES

The fear of SARS spreads faster than the virus. Older people in the wider community were very worried about SARS, especially those who lived alone, according to a local survey. Because of the avoidance of social contacts, they tended to stay at home, and social centers for the elderly were closed down. The avoidance of hospitals and doctors was even more marked. The hospital admission rates, attendance rates at public as well as private outpatient clinics, were all drastically reduced. On the other hand, the publicity about the "silent" older SARS patients reinforced the negative image of older people.

PREVENTION OF SARS IN THE FUTURE

Notwithstanding that the threat of SARS is fading, there is still a need to prevent the resurgence of the disease. The diagnostic difficulties of SARS in older people remain a concern, and may potentially spark off another outbreak, as in Toronto. The prevention of unnecessary hospital admission of older people, especially old-age home residents, by enhancing community medical and nursing support should be an important part of the overall preventive strategy.

SUMMARY

SARS in older people involves a high mortality rate. The clinical features of SARS in older people are more subtle and atypical. Cross infections in hospitals and old-age homes are important modes of transmission. Therefore, the prevention of unnecessary hospital admissions and enhanced medical surveillance in old-age homes are important in the prevention of the possible resurgence of SARS in older people.

FURTHER READING

Booth CM, Matukas LM, Tomlinson GA, *et al.* Clinical features and short term outcomes of 144 patients with SARS in the greater Toronto area. *JAMA* 2003;**289**:2861–3.

Donnelly CA, Ghani AC, Leung GM, *et al.* Epidemiological determinants of spread of causal agent of severe acute respiratory syndrome in Hong Kong. *Lancet* 2003;**361**:1761–6.

Lee N, Hui D, Wu A, *et al.* A major outbreak of severe acute respiratory syndrome in Hong Kong. *N Engl J Med* 2003;**348**:1986–94.

Position statement of the Hong Kong Geriatrics Society on Severe Acute Respiratory Syndrome (SARS) in Elders. http://medicine.org.hk/hkgs.

Rainer TH, Cameron PA, Smit D, *et al.* Evaluation of WHO criteria for identifying patients with severe acute respiratory syndrome out of hospital: prospective study. *BMJ* 2003;**326**:1354–62.

Riley S, Fraser C, Donnelly CA, *et al.* Transmission dynamics of the etiological agent of SARS in Hong Kong: impact of public health interventions. *Science* 2003;**300**:1961–6.

13

Severe Acute Respiratory Syndrome in Children

TF Fok

EPIDEMIOLOGY

Compared with that in adults, the prevalence of SARS was lower in children in the recent Hong Kong outbreak. Among the 1450 confirmed cases, only about 6% involved children less than 18 years of age. The age-specific prevalence rate was about 0.8% among children less than 14 years of age, which is significantly lower than those of the other age groups, which ranged from 2.0 to 7.7 per 10000 population.[1] There is no difference in attack rate between males and females. The youngest child confirmed to have SARS was 2 months of age. Most of the pediatric SARS cases have a positive history of close contact with one or more infected adults who are either household members or healthcare workers. Their infectivity appears to be significantly lower than that of the adult SARS patients. So far there has been no evidence of spread from children to children or from children to adults in the hospitals or the community. During the SARS outbreak in Hong Kong, although some of the pediatric SARS patients were attending school when they developed symptoms of the infection, there has been no evidence of spread of the infection in schools.[2]

CLINICAL FEATURES

The incubation period of SARS in children appears to be similar to that in adults, ranging from 3 to 11 days. The predominant symptoms are persistent fever, cough, malaise and coryza.[3] The clinical presentations and severity of the disease are related to the age of the patients.[2,4,5] The teenage patients present with symptoms similar to in adults, which include malaise, myalgia, chills and rigor. The younger children present mainly with cough and runny nose which are often indistinguishable from common cold or other types of viral upper respiratory tract infection. Chills, rigor and myalgia are notably absent. Asymptomatic cases with a history of close household contact with infected adults have been identified by serological test and viral studies of pharyngeal aspirates.

The severity and course of the illness also vary with age. In young children, the disease runs a mild course and most of the patients become afebrile within a week, and the triphasic pattern of the clinical course described in adults[6] is not observed. Only very few progress to respiratory distress and most do not require supplemental oxygen.[2,4,5] The pneumonic changes on chest radiographs are usually mild and usually disappear within two weeks of onset of symptoms.[4] Because of the mild nature of the disease, the use of the term "severe acute respiratory distress syndrome" in young children has been disputed. In contrast, the clinical course of adolescent patients is closer to in adults. They may show progressive deterioration over the first two weeks, with progressive respiratory distress and increase in oxygen supplementation.[2,4,5] Radiological changes are more profound than those in young children. The symptoms of the pediatric SARS patients reported in two published cohorts[4,5] are summarized in Table 1.

INVESTIGATIONS

The laboratory investigations of these patients are non-specific and often indistinguishable from those of other viral infections of the respiratory tract. Lymphopenia is a consistent feature, being present in over 90% of the patients.[2,4] Up to 40% to 50% of the patients have thrombocytopenia, which is usually mild.[2,4] Mild clotting derangement with prolonged prothrombin time and partial thromboplastin time, and elevated D-dimer may be present.[2,4] The most common biochemical derangement include

Table 1 Symptoms of 64 Confirmed SARS Cases admitted
into Princess Margaret Hospital[5] and United Christian
Hospital[4] during the SARS Outbreak in Hong Kong

Symptoms	No.	%
Fever	62	96.9
Malaise	38	59.4
Cough	37	57.7
Coryza	24	37.5
Chills and/or rigor	24	37.5
Sputum production	21	32.9
Myalgia	18	28.1
Headache	18	28.1
Anorexia	15	23.4
Dizziness	13	20.3
Diarrhea	9	14.1
Sore throat	8	12.5
Dyspnea	7	10.9

elevated serum lactic dehydrogenase and creatine phosphokinase levels, which affected 71.4% and 42.9% of the infected children in one series.[4]

All the children have pneumonic changes on chest radiographs.[4] Some children may have normal chest X-ray on admission but develop radiological changes during the course of the illness. The primary abnormality is airspace opacification. There may be focal segmental consolidation or ill defined patchy consolidation which may be unilateral or bilateral. Despite clinical improvement, these consolidative changes often persist into the second week but usually resolve completely within 14 days. In some patients, chest radiographs taken at the early stage of the illness may not reveal any abnormality, but high resolution CT thorax may demonstrate the presence of focal consolidations and characteristic features of peripheral and alveolar opacities simulating the radiological features of bronchiolitis obliterans organizing pneumonia.[2]

Detection of the RNA of coronavirus in nasopharyngeal aspirate using reversed transcriptase-polymerase chain reaction has been employed for the rapid diagnosis of SARS, but the method has not proven to be of sufficient sensitivity. The condition is most reliably diagnosed by serological method. However, a significant rise in the coronavirus neutralizing antibody level takes place fairly late in the course of the disease, often up to 21 days after onset of symptoms.

TREATMENT

During the SARS outbreak in Hong Kong, a treatment protocol has been jointly formulated by the pediatricians from the Prince of Wales Hospital and Princess Margaret Hospital, which were the hospitals that admitted the earliest cases of pediatric SARS patients.[7] In this protocol, children who satisfy the following criteria will be treated as suspected SARS cases:

1. Fever (rectal temperature ≥38.5°C or oral temperature ≥38°C); and
2. Contact with a person under investigation for or diagnosed with SARS, or exposure to a locality with suspected or documented community transmission of SARS, either through travel or residence, with 10 days of onset of symptoms; and
3. Presence of one or more of the following: chills, malaise, myalgia, muscle fatigue, cough, dyspnea, tachypnea, or non-response of fever to antibiotics covering the usual pathogens of community acquired pneumonia after two days of therapy.

All suspected SARS cases were given a combination of antibiotics (a third generation cephalosporin such as cefotaxime, and a macrolide such as Clarithromycin) to cover for the common bacterial and atypical pneumonia. This is important since a number of children with bacterial sepsis have been diagnosed with suspected SARS at first presentation. Oral ribavirin were also be started at a dose of 40–60 mg/kg/d in three divided doses. If fever persisted for two days and there was deterioration or no improvement in general well being, oral prednisolone were commenced at a dose of 1–2 mg/kg/d in two divided doses (or intravenous hydrocortisone 1–2 mg/kg 6 hourly). If there was progressive deterioration clinically or on chest radiographs, methylprednisolone 10 mg/kg/dose will be given every 24 h for up to 3 doses. Ribavirin would also be changed to the intravenous form (20–30 mg/kg/d in 3 divided doses).

Systemic antibiotics was discontinued if the child had been afebrile for five days. Ribavirin was given for a total of 10–14 days. Use of prednisolone or hydrocortisone would taper off after 1–2 weeks of treatment, depending on the rate of improvement and resolution of pneumonic changes on chest X-ray.

OUTCOME AND PROGNOSIS

Compared with adult SARS, the disease appears to be a much milder condition in the pediatric age group. In the recent Hong Kong outbreak, there is not a single case of fatality among the pediatric patients. The condition is particularly mild in the young children and often indistinguishable from other kinds of mild viral infection despite the presence of pneumonic changes on chest radiographs. Although the symptoms in adolescent patients are more similar to those in adults, very few required intensive care even in this group, and only one a teenage girl required intubation and mechanical ventilation.[5] It is not known whether the milder nature of the disease in children is related to differences in their immunological reaction to the virus when compared with that in adults. Whether the infection will lead to any long term sequelae on the pulmonary function or airway hyper-reactivity of the children has also yet to be determined.

BABIES BORN TO SARS MOTHERS[8]

Five babies were born to mothers confirmed to have SARS during the outbreak in Hong Kong. Four were preterm infants born at gestations of 26, 28, 32, and 33 weeks, respectively. The fifth one was born at 37 weeks of gestation. In addition to complications of prematurity, including respiratory distress syndrome, both extremely preterm infants developed intestinal perforation due to necrotizing enterocolitis in one, and clean perforation in the other. Both were delivered by emergency Caesarean section because of rapid deterioration of the mothers' condition. RT-PCR study of their peritoneal fluid did not show the presence of the SARS coronavirus. Antenatally, both mothers had experienced hypoxic or hypotensive episodes, and had been treated with high dose pulsed methylprednisolone. It is not known how much these events have contributed to the intestinal complication. Exhaustive virological studies including RT-PCR study on placental swab, urine, serum, endotracheal aspirate, pernasal swab, throat swab, gastric fluid, stool, and cerebrospinal fluid, and serological test were all negative for the SARS coronavirus. Their clinical features, hematological and biochemical studies also showed no features of SARS. It thus appears that infants born to mothers infected with SARS are not necessarily infected.

REFERENCES

1. University of Hong Kong Centre of Clinical Trial. University of Hong Kong Centre of Clinical Trial Web Site. http://www.hku.hk/ctc/index.htm 2003.

2. Hon KLE, Leung CW, Cheng WTF, *et al.* Clinical presentations and outcome of severe acute respiratory syndrome in children. *Lancet* 2003;http://image.thelancet.com/extras/03let4127web.pdf.

3. Wong GWK, Li AM, Ng PC, Fok TF. Severe acute respiratory syndrome in children. *Pediatr Pulmonol* 2003;**36**:1–6.

4. Chiu WK, Cheung PCH, Ng KL, *et al.* Severe acute respiratory syndrome in children: Experience in a regional hospital in Hong Kong. *Pediatr Crit Care Med* 2003;**4**(279):83.

5. Leung CW. Clinical features, diagnosis, treatment and short-term outcome of severe acute respiratory syndrome (SARS) in children. *HK J Paediatr* 2003;**8**:245–7.

6. Lee N, Hui D, Wu A, *et al.* A major outbreak of severe acute respiratory syndrome in Hong Kong. NEJM 2003; http://content.nejm.org/cgi/reprint/NEJMoa030685v2.pdf.

7. Leung CW, Li CK. PMH/PWH interim guidelines on the management of children with SARS. *HK J Paediatr* 2003;**8**:168–9.

8. Shek CC, Ng PC, Fung GPG, *et al.* Infants born to mothers with severe acute respiratory syndrome. *Pediatrics* 2003;**112**:e254–e256.

14

Nursing Management of Severe Acute Respiratory Syndrome

David R Thompson, Violeta Lopez

INTRODUCTION

The recent outbreak of a new infectious disease, severe acute respiratory syndrome (SARS), has had a major impact on nurses and nursing care. This chapter aims to provide a concise and up-to-date overview of the nursing management of patients with SARS and to highlight the major clinical, educational and public health implications.

NURSING MANAGEMENT

As SARS is a new disease, the nursing management of patients with SARS depends largely on their clinical presentation and on the day-to-day evaluation of their condition. Nursing management will continue to change as new information becomes available.[1] But a major goal is to provide physical care and psychological support based on a systematic and thorough assessment of the patients' needs as well as tailored to individual circumstances. Nursing aims to prevent the disease from spreading, reduce risk and promote health.

Table 1   Documentation for Suspected and Probable Cases of SARS

Surveillance and Monitoring Forms	Content
SARS Reporting Form (Appendix 1)	Case definition information, biographical and medical history as well as history of travel outside Hong Kong within 30 days of onset of symptoms
Initial Screening Form (Appendix 2)	Symptoms associated with SARS
Reassessment Form (Appendix 2)	Day-to-day progress, discharge and diagnosis
Investigation, Treatment and Progress Form (Appendix 3)	Investigation results, specific medications, complications, progress and plan

Surveillance and Monitoring

Surveillance and monitoring forms have been developed by the Hospital Authority (HA) in Hong Kong to be used by all hospitals admitting suspected and probable cases of SARS, as shown in Table 1. In addition, individual hospitals have produced their own more detailed forms for investigation, treatment and progress of patients with SARS.

Nurses must complete the registry of new cases of SARS, gather important information about the patient's history and response to treatment, and record discharges and deaths. These records could serve as a database that aids understanding of the forms of transmissibility and also to monitor the virus response to therapy.

Probable and suspected cases of SARS need to be admitted to SARS designated wards, and nurses must be vigilant in monitoring the patients' condition. Routine vital signs and other hemodynamic parameters, including oxygen saturation and urine output, should be monitored and recorded accurately on the observations charts. Any adverse effects to ribavirin, corticosteroids and nutritional feeds should also be monitored and reported promptly.[2]

Infection Control

A key aspect of nursing management is infection control. Early recognition and isolation of patients with SARS is vital due to the high infectivity of the SARS-CoV. Given that the mode of transmission of the SARS virus

is usually by droplet, it is important to take appropriate isolation precautions with patients suspected with SARS, with guidance from the
Centers for Disease Control and Prevention (CDC) and the World Health
Organization (WHO) (see http://.cdc.gov.ncidod.sars.ic.htm and http://
www.who.int/csr/sars/ic.htm, respectively). Isolation of patients suspected of having SARS in a negative-pressure room is recommended
when feasible. Otherwise, categorizing clinical areas as a SARS-
designated ward may help reduce cross contamination. However, one of
the challenges in reducing cross contamination is the basic failing of
many existing healthcare facilities, including overcrowded wards, poor
ventilation, lack of isolation facilities, and staff working under stressful
conditions. Such failing could be prevented by planning workflow
patterns, consulting hospital engineers to improve ventilation and
increasing distances between patients' beds.

Nurses should ensure that infection control protocols are in line with
the CDC recommendations for isolation precautions in hospitals (see
http://www.cdc.gov/ncidod/hip/ISOLAT/isopart2.htm), particularly
those recommendations pertaining to droplet transmission. Infection control measures include the use of personal protective equipment (PPE) of
which a N-95 mask, gloves, caps, and disposable protective apparel or
gown, goggles/visors and/or face shields are used during direct patient
contact. Although the use of PPE is recommended, in clinical practice it is
not without its challenges, not least in posing a barrier to the nurse-
patient relationship. For example, the wearing of N-95 mask is not only
uncomfortable but inhibits effective communication and limits personal
human contact with patients and relatives. Also, nurses often have difficulty in obtaining a mask that fits correctly and thus affords maximum
protection. Wearing full protective gear limits freedom of movement,
causes sweating and overheating and, if not changed/replaced regularly,
may induce concerns about its efficacy in offering protection. PPE is only
effective if used correctly and does not replace basic hygiene measures.
For example, the wearing of gloves does not replace the need for thorough hand washing. The practice of droplet precaution and frequent
hand washing may be the most important measures to reduce the risks of
nosocomial transmission of the SARS virus from one person or site to
another.[3]

Staff should be properly trained in the correct use and removal of
PPE and reminded of the importance of hand hygiene. The safety and

effectiveness of reusable PPE depends on its proper usage and maintenance. Therefore, all users must receive training and each clinical area should have a designated person responsible for the maintenance and disinfection of PPE. Documented training on infection control should be mandatory. The infection control team should establish PPE standards, making reference to the recommended minimum standards by authoritative bodies.

To safeguard the health of all patients, staff and members of the public, visitors must be restricted in acute wards and prohibited from visiting their relatives in the intensive care unit. Visiting relatives, if allowed by the healthcare facility, should be kept to a minimum, and should be issued with protective equipment, educated on infection control measures and must be supervised. Visitors who have symptoms of fever, cough and/or diarrhea are advised not to visit and to seek medical treatment. The hospital may require visitors to complete a form to enable contact tracing.

All staff caring for SARS patients should adopt precautionary measures at home for at least 10 days from the latest contact with SARS patients. These precautionary measures include: frequent hand-washing with liquid soap; putting on surgical masks; avoiding sharing of food and eating utensils and towels; avoiding close contact such as kissing and hugging; and maintaining good home ventilation.

Disinfectants such as quaternary ammonium-based, phenol-based, and alcohol-based products are considered active against SARS-CoV[4] and must be used for environmental and equipment cleaning. Recent data suggest that the virus may remain viable for considerable periods on dry surfaces for up to 24 hours. Frequent surface cleansing of the clinical areas should be enforced, such as the use of a 1 in 49 dilution of hypochlorite for non-metallic and 70% alcohol solution for metallic items. Surfaces contaminated with vomitus, blood, excreta should be immediately disinfected with a 1 in 5 dilution of hypochlorite solution. Soiled linens should be disposed off as clinical waste. Staff involved in cleaning the clinical areas and equipment should undergo infection control training and must understand the importance of adhering to the infection control guidelines. Amenities (e.g. pens and paper) should not be brought in and out of the SARS clinical area, and eating within the confines of the clinical area must be prohibited.

The rate of deterioration of patients with SARS may be high with many requiring intensive care due to severe desaturation and worsening lung damage in spite of oxygen therapy. This may result in patients requiring tracheal intubation and mechanical ventilation to correct the ventilation-perfusion mismatch. Because the main mode of transmission of the virus is by droplet, treatment with a nebulizer and the use of noninvasive positive pressure ventilation is avoided in patients with fever and chest X-ray infiltrates. The use of high-flow Venturi masks should also be avoided because the high flow could facilitate dissemination of droplets when the patient coughs. For mechanically ventilated patients, a bacterial/viral filter is connected to the breathing circuit. A closed-suction system is also used to prevent breaking of the ventilator circuit when suctioning the patient is carried out. All equipment used must be disposed off in a clearly marked contaminated bag and disposed off or sterilized accordingly.

Nutritional Support

Gastrointestinal functions are affected under stress especially in patients who require mechanical ventilation. Malnutrition could become a problem in most critically ill patients and, therefore, nutritional support is required. The decision with regard to the type of feeding patients receives depends on the assessment of the patients' nutritional needs and biochemical data. The Hospital Authority of Hong Kong has outlined a set of guidelines in terms of a feeding regimen through either an oral, enteral or parenteral route. Nurses must ensure that patients are receiving the right amount of feeds and monitor for complications associated with malabsorption such as diarrhea. When severe diarrhea occurs, patients are given anti-diarrheal drug therapy. A rectal tube may be inserted to contain the watery stools of patients. Normally, the insertion of rectal tube is no longer advocated due to the associated risk of complications. However, this practice is used in SARS as evidence also shows that SARS-CoV in feces could be a source of infection.[5] Diarrhea is also a common complication of antibiotic therapy. Nurses should also collect stool specimens for microbiological testing.

Prevention of Complications

In mechanically ventilated patients, nurses should monitor them for cardiac and lung complications. Cardiac complications include hypotension and fluid retention. Hypotension is caused by the application of positve pressure ventilation with high positive end expiratory pressure (PEEP), which increases intrathoracic pressure and inhibiting blood return to the heart. Fluid retention occurs due to decreased cardiac output. In addition, the lungs experience barotraumas (e.g. pneumothorax or subcutaneous emphysema), volutrauma and acid-base abnormalities. Cardiopulmonary (vital signs and chest auscultation) and renal (hourly urine output) assessments must be performed to monitor these complications, so that prompt corrective interventions can be instituted. In some cases, patients may develop a bilateral pneumothorax and a chest drain will need to be inserted. Careful monitoring of patients with chest drains connected to an underwater sealed drainage system must be maintained. Other patients may require continuous venovenous hemofiltration with dialysis (CVVHD) to correct renal dysfunction. The hospital protocol for the management of patients on CVVHD should be followed and should include careful monitoring of electrolyte levels and for complications such as hypovolemia, hypotension/hypertension and dysrrhythmias.

Muscular deconditioning can also occur because of prolonged immobility. Assisting the patient to rehabilitate early and to perform exercises can improve muscle tone and strength. However, patients who are critically ill and those who are mechanically ventilated and receiving muscle relaxants will need passive muscle exercises on a routine basis. Such nursing activity improves muscle tone and strength, facilitates gas exchange and promotes oxygen delivery to all muscles. Exercise may also prevent the development of deep venous thrombosis of the legs. Patients are also fitted with graded elastic stockings and given a prophylactic dose of low molecular weight heparin intravenously to prevent deep venous thrombosis.

Patient/Family Education

Health education will play a significant role in containing the spread of the disease in the community. Strategies will need to be targeted at individuals, whether at home or work, in terms of personal hygiene and lifestyle to ensure that people maximize their level of immunity.

Prior to discharge, patients must be told to stay away from work, school or other activities in a public place for 10 days after resolution of fever. When discharged home, household members must be advised to wear disposable gloves and practice good hand washing when having direct contact with body fluids of the recuperating person. The sharing of eating utensils, towels and bedding should be avoided. Household contact should be reported to the hospital if anyone develops a fever or respiratory symptoms.[6]

Psychological Support

SARS is extremely distressing for the patient as well as their family. Patients are likely to feel highly anxious and they will require an assessment of their psychological state. Anxiety is common and can be minimized if information tailored to their needs is given to patients. Effective communication is central to information giving. Reassurance and preparation for unpleasant procedures can help alleviate anxiety by removing the additional burden of facing the unknown.[7]

Depression can range from mild to severe and from transient to persistent. Education, advice and reassurance that involve the patients and their partners or other key family members are often beneficial.[8] The screening and management of anxiety and depression is essential and the development of a treatment plan should be based on systematic assessment.

Once patients with SARS are admitted to hospital, strict isolation means that relatives are not permitted to visit so as to prevent them from contracting the disease. This has to be handled sensitively in order to avoid frustration and isolation of patients from their loved ones. To overcome such problems, a telephone link up should be established to permit contact, boost morale and alleviate distress. Also, where appropriate, counseling, debriefing and monitoring of progress are essential.

Support for staff in terms of professional guidance and an opportunity for sharing of views and experiences is crucial.[9] In order to support them, the establishment of a counseling "hot-line" and the provision of intensive training and preceptorship programs for new nurses working with SARS patients are likely to be beneficial.

Public Health Implications

SARS has an enormous impact on the community as well as public health. Community and public health nurses will need to ensure that good communication systems, such as a website, are established and that appropriate and timely information that outlines strategies to prevent the spread of the disease is produced and circulated.[1] However, procedures such as contact tracing and quarantining of suspected contacts will also need to be implemented.

SARS indicates a reaffirmation of the importance of health promotion to the health of the community. The importance of the partnership of public health policy and health education cannot be stressed too much. Policy implications may include the cleansing of public areas and the enforcement of building regulations. At a more micro-level, policies must be in place to ensure that all schools make available liquid soap in toilets for use by the children. The school health nurses must be knowledgeable of the mode of transmission of the SARS virus and continue to educate not only the school children but also all school teachers and parents. This is important to ensure that personal hygiene of school children is carried out not only within the school grounds but also at home.

The outbreak of SARS has also brought various psychological reactions from the public. A recent study has shown that nearly 80% of the 1002 members of the public surveyed were worried about the spread of the disease to the community; 40% felt scared and helpless about its spread; and 20% were concerned about contracting the disease.[10] It is recommended that vigorous public health education programs should be launched to enhance the public's understanding of the disease and the adoption of preventative health measures against SARS.

Organizational Implications

One of the lessons of SARS is the ability of nurses and nursing to mobilize their expertise and resources at short notice to deal creatively with an unexpected health emergency.[9] During the initial outbreak of SARS, concerns were raised by frontline clinical nurses about the lack of communication and the ineffective dissemination of information, in particular, regarding their role during this outbreak. The deployment of nurses to a SARS-designated ward and intensive care unit requires them to be more flexible and responsive in such situations, acknowledging that this might be discomfiting and difficult at times. The organization has the responsibility to provide intensive training and preceptorship to these nurses. Training could be organized using on-line teaching or a more traditional classroom approach to teaching and learning. The initial training must be followed by clinical supervision using the preceptorship model, wherein novice nurses are supervised by experienced ones in the clinical area. The continuing education of all nurses about SARS should be the norm, so that nurses working in non-SARS-designated areas are prepared for possible deployment and prompt identification of suspected cases. Nurse managers should shoulder the responsibility for ensuring that continuing education is provided as this is a key to promoting and maintaining competency and improving patient care quality.

Educational Implications

The education of the next generation of nurses will now take into account what was learned from the SARS outbreak. The nursing curriculum needs to be revisited in terms of its content and timing of delivery in relation to infection control measures.[1] It is imperative that sufficient time and importance be devoted to the topic early in the nursing curriculum as a prerequisite to being exposed to patients. In addition, in the final-year the mandatory completion of an infection control module seems sensible. This will not only serve as a reminder of the nurse's professional responsibility and a clinical update, but also afford optimal protection to patients, relatives and themselves.

CONCLUSION

The nursing management of patients with SARS necessitates a systematic assessment of individual needs and the planning, implementation and evaluation of evidence-based care. Infection control measures will need to be implemented and strictly adhered to. Isolation and quarantine measures may be warranted in some circumstances. Attention to the psychological state of patients and family members and the provision of appropriate support should not be overlooked. Patient and family education is paramount to the whole enterprise. Nurses also play a crucial role in the detection, containment and prevention of SARS.

REFERENCES

1. Thompson DR, Lopez V, Lee D, Twinn S. SARS — A perspective from a school of nursing in Hong Kong. *J Clin Nurs* 2004;**13**:131–135.

2. Lopez V, Chan KS, Wong YC. Nursing care of patients with Severe Acute Respiratory Syndrome in the intensive care unit: Case reports in Hong Kong. *Int J Nur Studies* 2004;**41**:263–272.

3. Seto WH, Tsang D, Yung RWH, *et al.* Effectiveness of precautions against droplets and contact in prevention of nosocomial transmission of severe acute respiratory syndrome (SARS). *Lancet* 2003; **361**:1519–1520.

4. Wenzel RP, Edmund M. Managing SARS amidst uncertainty. *N Eng J Med* 2003;**348**:1947–1948.

5. Drosten C, Gunther S, Preiser W, *et al.* Identification of a novel SARS-CoV in patients with severe acute respiratory syndrome. *N Eng J Med* 2003;**348**:1967–1976.

6. Sampathkumar P, Temesgen Z, Smith TF, Thompson RL. SARS: Epidemiology, clinical manifestations, management and infection control measures. *Mayo Clin Proc* 2003;**78:** 882–890.

7. House A, Stark D. Anxiety in medical patients. *B M J* 2002;**325**: 207–209.

8. Peveler R, Carson A, Rodin G. Depression in medical patients. *B M J* 2002;**325**:149–152.

9. Thompson DR. SARS — Some lessons for nursing. *J Clin Nurs* 2003; **12**:615–617.

10. Tang CSK, Wong JCY. Survey results on public responses to atypical pneumonia in Hong Kong. Accessed July 18, 2003 at http://www.cuhk.edu.hk/ipro/pressrelease/030320e.htm.

SARS Reporting Form, Hospital Authority

To be completed by chest physician, infectious disease physician or ICU physician

CONFIDENTIAL

Case Definition of SARS (Revision date: 22/3/2003)
Inclusion:
4.   Presence of new radiological infiltrates compatible with pneumonia, and
5.   Fever ≥ 38°C, or history of such any time in the last 2 days, and
6.   At least 2 of the following:
a.   Chills any time in the last 2 days
b.   New or increased cough
c.   General malaise
d.   Typical physical signs of consolidation
If no known history of exposure, consider exclusion if presence of any one of:
4.   Leucocytosis on admission
5.   CXR show lobar consolidation
6.   The pathogen is already known

How to report?

(i)   **Input data directly into the HA SARS Registry (for those with program installed), or**

(ii)   **Complete this form & fax to 28815848 and 27720917**

From: _____ Hospital   Date of Report: _____

(dd/mm/yy)

(No need to enter if gum label is available)	
HKID / Passport no.	
Sex Age	
Date of Admission	

Circle the correct choice(s), select more than one if indicated.

Date of onset:	Symptom:	Fever ≥38°C:
History of Contact with probable SARS:	Yes / No Source:_____ _____ _____ *Surname* *Full Name* *HKID (if available)* Place of contact: Exposure date: Nature of contact:	
Does any family member or close contact has symptom?	Yes / No Specify:	
History of Travel outside HK within 30 days of onset of symptoms:	Yes / No Destination city: Date(s):	
Occupation	Healthcare worker (Doctor / Nurse / Allied Health / HCA / Lab staff / Other: _____) Non-health care worker:	
Daytime address (if different from home, e.g. company, school, old age home, etc.)	Institute / Building: District:	
Underlying chronic disease	Yes / No	
On admission	Overall condition	Stable / Respiratory distress / ICU
	Body temperature	
	CXR	
Condition on report day	Discharged / Stable / Respiratory distress / ICU / Died	
Any other relevant information		

Appendix 2

Part A   Initial Screening (Day 0)

_____   Undifferentiated febrile illness
_____   Likely bacterial / lobar pneumonia
_____   Likely atypical pneumonia, no risk factor
_____   *Likely atypical pneumonia, high risk case**
(*single room isolation if available*)

   * *high risk case: family clustering, contact with known or highly suspicious case.*

Part B   Reassessment

	Day 1	Day 2	Day 3	Day 4	Day 5	Day 6	Day 7	Day 8	Day 9	Day 10	Day 11	Day 12
Same as Part A												
Influenza A												
Influenza B												
Viral syndrome, undifferentiated												
Viral pneumonia – Inf A												
Viral pneumonia – Inf B												
Atypical pneumonia, undifferentiated, no risk factor												
Atypical pneumonia high risk*												
Bacterial pneumonia												
TB												
Infection in other organ (Dx _____)												
Improving												
Static												
Worsening												
Keep in cohort area												
Keep single room isolation												
Off cohorting, droplets precaution												
Discharge												

* *High risk case: family clustering, contact with known or highly suspicious case.*

Final diagnosis and aetiological agent: 1) _____
                                           2) _____
                                           3) _____

182

Treatment and Progress Report

Date: Time:

Background Information		Investigation Result
Name		RT-PCR
Sex		Stool-PCR
Occupation		G6PD
Date of onset of symptoms		HbsAg
DOA to Hospital		HCV
DOA to ICU		Serology on 1st on titre
Ventilated since		2nd on titre
		3rd on titre

Treatment

                                        start on   stopped on

Ribarivin

Pulse Methylprednisolone

                    Total dosage

Levofloxacin

Doxycycline

Tazocin

Maxipime

Pavulon

LMWH

Complications:

Pneumomediastinum

DVT

Progress

CXR

Fever

I/O Balance

Diarrhoea

Urea

CRP

Hb   Platelet

WBC

Plan

15

Herbal Medicine in the Treatment of SARS

PC Leung

Whether the recent SARS epidemic originated in the Pearl Delta in the Guangdong province of China or elsewhere was not entirely clear. However, that the first case of SARS in China occurred in the Pearl Delta region, and which later spread to Guangzhou, Hong Kong and Beijing was an officially accepted fact. It was observed that the mortality rate of SARS in China was apparently lower than those in other countries, including Hong Kong, Toronto and Singapore. It had been revealed in the media, throughout the SARS outbreak, that Chinese physicians were applying an integrated approach, using both modern medicine and herbs, in the treatment of SARS. It was, therefore, assumed that this integrated approach had brought down the mortality rate.

The traditional use of Chinese herbal medicine for the treatment of diseases is very much a cultural activity widely valued by the people of Chinese descent. It is therefore easy to find enthusiastic supporters; on the other hand, skepticism is not usually expressed openly.[1] In order to evaluate the efficacy of herbal medicine, reliable scientific clinical data from China are required, including the actual number of patients treated using this approach, details of treatment, the timing, and how the patients' responses differed from those in the conventional groups. It is also necessary to look at the indications of treatment selection, whether the approach was a full scale integration, or only a partial one. Without these data, the experience could not be properly evaluated. One could not simply assume that the use of Chinese medicine has led to improved survival of the patients with SARS based on media reports alone.

VIEWS OF THE MINISTRY OF HEALTH OF CHINA

The Centre for the Prevention and Control of Diseases under the Ministry of Health of China has issued special instructions and guidelines to the hospitals and clinics on special disease conditions and their diagnoses and treatments. Such guidelines are quite specific and detailed.

In early 2003, when atypical pneumonia started to spread in Southern China, the information gathered was scattered. The etiology and clinical presentations of the infection were not properly reported and professional analyses were disappointing. There was, therefore, the assumption that the causative agent was neither a bacterium nor a virus, but a rare clamydium.[2]

In April 2003, the Centre gathered all the available information from both inside and outside China, gave an updated analysis, and revised the deduction on the SARS outbreak. A complete set of documents, containing details of etiology, diagnostic criteria, clinical manifestations, management, instructions, drugs used, preventive means and Chinese medicinal considerations was produced.[3]

Concerning Chinese medicine, the Centre labeled SARS as a form of Wan Bing (温病). Wan Bing, meaning diseases with temperature, was an important specialization within Traditional Chinese Medicine. Although diseases with increased body temperature were described and well documented more than 2000 years ago in the Han Dynasty, when Zhang Zhon-jing (張仲景), one of the forefathers of Chinese medicine, wrote his book "Shang-han Luen" (傷寒論),[4] and although the classic volume had been taken as a detailed documentation on typhoid, the descriptions in reality, exceeded the realm of typhoid. It encompassed a much larger area of diseases of probably infectious nature. Followers of Zhang refined and expanded the understanding of the specialty during the dynasties following Han. A clear-cut and well recognized specialty of Wan Bing finally matured in the years between the Ming and Qing Dynasties. It is not an exaggeration to consider this specialty as the most important branch of Chinese Herbal Medicine, covering the most frequently encountered areas of the herbalist's practice, commanding numerous volumes of case reports and prescriptions and above all, it has been included in the teaching curricula of all educational set-ups on Chinese medicine and considered mandatory.[5]

A term coined using the common language of everyday use, Wan Bing was understood as referring to the common, feverish diseases appearing at the intervals between weather changes, i.e. between spring and summer, and between autumn and winter. These feverish diseases were contagious, first spreading within the family household, later spreading outside to the village; and later, even across villages.

Having labeled the current SARS outbreak as a form of Wan Bing, the Centre for Diseases Control and Prevention recommended treatment protocols, according to the Wan Bing classical teaching. With regard to hospitalized patients, the Centre's guidelines for treatment include the following:[3]

(1) Use antibiotics to prevent bacterial infection,
(2) Consider using steroidal preparations to control excessive immunological responses,
(3) Consider using herbal preparations as an adjuvant therapy, and
(4) Use antiviral preparations.

One month later, in an updated version, the Centre revised the order of the instructions, elevating the use of antiviral preparations from the fourth to the third position.[6]

From the Official, National guidelines on the treatment of SARS, it was obvious that as far as hospitalized patients were concerned, modern medicine remained the mainstream treatment and Chinese medicine was used a supportive, adjuvant therapy. There were no instructions on the use of herbal medicine in the management of SARS during the early, pre-hospitalized stage or the later convalescent, rehabilitation stage.

MANAGEMENT OF SARS PATIENTS IN THE HOSPITALS IN CHINA

If there were official reports describing the precise hospital management of SARS patients with or without Chinese herbal supplements, they should be good references. However, since such comprehensive documents were not available, we had to rely on media accounts, documentations, conferences and personal knowledge.

One has to understand that although some hospitals in China were named "Chinese Medicine Hospital", it does not mean that only Chinese medicine is being given as the agent for healing. In fact, the so-called Chinese Medicine Hospitals fulfill the duties of any other hospitals, i.e. catering to emergencies, intensive care and invasive means of rescue, like modern investigations, surgeries and other interventions. The only difference, unique to Chinese Medicine Hospital, is that Chinese medicine use is always considered, whenever treatment is being offered. When SARS patients were admitted into Chinese Medicine Hospitals, therefore, herbal medicine would be used as part of the treatment regime. As for the other hospitals, whether Chinese medicine would be included as adjuvant therapy; it would depend on the attending team of physicians and the patients and their relatives. Only about 10% of the hospitals in China carried the hallmark of Chinese Medicine Hospital and were functionally Chinese Medicine Hospitals.[7]

Based on these facts, an estimated 40–60% of hospitalized SARS patients at some stages of their treatment, received an integrated approach, combining both modern and Chinese medicine. This was confirmed by the Deputy Minister of Health of Municipal Beijing towards the end stage of the SARS outbreak.[8]

My personal contacts from the hospitals in Guangzhou and Beijing have also informed me that the overall situation in the Infections Hospitals and hospitals assigned to deal with the SARS crisis, had a similar offer to patients. Usually, where *responses* were straightforward, only modern medicine would be given. When responses were not satisfactory, especially at the requests of relatives, an integrated approach would be applied. Unfortunately, very often, the integrated approach was started too late. In fact, earlier, we have heard respiratory physicians in China making negative comments like "the conceptual use of herbal medicine in SARS management", which could be quite disturbing for the advocates of the integrated approach.

Positive reports, on the other hand, were quite plentiful. A professor from Shanghai visited the Chinese Medicine University in Guangzhou in early June 2003, and reported that the first affiliated hospital of the University treated 60 patients with SARS, and the mortality rate was zero.

The second affiliated hospital treated double the number of SARS patients, and the mortality rate was only 6%, well below the data known for SARS infection outside China. Furthermore, it was reported that the hospital workers took prophylactic herbal drinks and none of them fell sick in spite of the high risk nature of their work.[2]

More detailed information about the treatment regimes as revealed in a teleconference between Taiwanese experts and Beijing physicians during the peak of the outbreak in Taiwan.[3] Apart from emphasizing the effectiveness of herbal medicine as an adjuvant therapy for SARS patients, and the need to properly utilize oxygen therapy, respirators, and steroids, a number of injection solutions manufactured from herbs were recommended to facilitate rapid interventional supplements. They were Qing Kai Ling (清開靈), a proprietor injection preparation; Herba Houttuyniae (魚腥草), Radix Isatidis (板藍根), and Xiangdian (香丹), another proprietor mixture.

As prophylaxis, six prescriptions were given. They were:-

(i)   Formula 1: 黄芪, 敗醬草, 薏苡仁, 桔梗, 生甘草.

(ii) Formula 2: 魚腥草, 野菊花, 茵陳, 佩蘭, 草果.

(iii) Formula 3: 蒲公英, 金蓮花, 大青葉, 葛根, 蘇葉.

(iv) Formula 4: 蘆根, 銀花, 連翹, 薄荷, 生甘草.

(v)   Formula 5: 黄芪, 白朮, 防風, 蒼朮, 藿香, 沙參, 銀花, 綿馬貫眾.

(vi) Formula 6: 太子參, 綿馬貫眾, 銀花, 連翹, 大青葉, 蘇葉,
      葛根, 藿香, 蒼朮, 佩蘭.

Formula	Herb Components		Botanical Name
1	黄芪	Huangqi	Radix Astragalus
	敗醬草	Paichiangtsao	Herba Patriniae
	薏苡仁	Yiyiren	Semen Coicis
	桔梗	Jiegeng	Radix Platycodonis
	甘草	Gnacao	Radix Glycyrrhizae
2	魚腥草	Yuxingcao	Herba Houttuyniae
	野菊花	Yrjhuhua	Flos Chrysanthemi Indici
	茵陳	Yinchen	Herba Artemisiae Scopariae
	佩蘭	Peilan	Herba Eupatorii
	草果	Caoguo	Fructus Tsaoko
3	蒲公英	Pugongying	Herba Taraxaci
	蓮花	Lian Hua	*Nelumbo nucifera* Gaerth.

Continued

	大青葉	Daqingye	Folium Isatidis
	葛根	Gegen	Radix Puerariae
	蘇葉	Suyeh	Folium Perillae
4	葦根	Lugen	Rhizoma Phragmitis
	金銀花	Jinyinhua	Lonicerae Flos
	連翹	Lienchiao	Fructus Forsythiae
	薄荷	Bohe	Herba Menthae
	甘草	Gnacao	Radix Glycyrrhizae
5	黃芪	Huangqi	Radix Astragalus
	白朮	Baizhu	Rhizoma Atractylodis Macrocephalae
	防風	Fangfeng	Radix Saposhnikoviae
	蒼朮	Cangzhu	Rhizoma Atractylodis
	藿香	Hohsiang	Herba Agastachis
	沙參	Sha Shen	*Adenophora stricta* Miq.
	金銀花	Jinyinhua	Lonicerae Flos
	綿馬貫眾	Mianmaguanzhoung	Rhizoma Dryopteris Crassihizomae
6	太子參	Taitaizishen	Radix Pseudostellariae
	綿馬貫眾	Mianmaguanzhoung	Rhizoma Dryopteris Crassirhizomae
	金銀花	Jinyinhua	Lonicerae Flos
	連翹	Lienchiao	Fructus Forsythiae
	大青葉	Daqingye	Folium Isatidis
	蘇葉	Suyeh	Folium Perillae
	葛根	Gegen	Radix Puerariae
	藿香	Hohsiang	Herba Agastachis
	蒼朮	Cangzhu	Rhizoma Atractylodis
	佩蘭	Peilan	Herba Eupatorii

Normally, herbal experts would advocate the individualization of prescriptions depending on circumstantial manifestations. However, as a prevention, more generalizations are allowed. Fixed prescriptions are feasible for the prophylactic treatment or treatment at the very early stages of the SARS infection.

When these formulae are carefully studied, they are found to resemble conventional recommendations for different situations of Wan Bing, with addition or subtraction of some herbs. These formulae are readily available in Wan Bing classics.

During the convalescent period when patients are weak and frail, their relatives and friends would know how to serve them with herbal preparations. One such formula was recommended by the National Institute on the Control of Chinese Medicine, labeled as "anti-fibrotic lung tonic". The herbs are as follows:

黃芪	Huangqi	Radix Astragalus
甘草	Gnacao	Radix Glycyrrhizae
太子參	Taizishen	Radix Pseudostellariae
五味子	Wuweizi	Fructus Schisandrae Chinensis
丹參	Danshen	Radix Salviae Miltiorrhizae
川芎	Chuanxiong	Rhizoma Chuanxiong
沙參	Shashen	Adenophora Stricta
天花粉	Tianhuafen	Radix Trichosanthis
麥冬	Maitung	Radix Ophiopogonis
桃仁	Taojen	Semen Persicae
半夏		Rhizoma Pinelliae

After the successful control of the SARS outbreak in Hong Kong and China, a conference was held at the Polytechnic University of Hong Kong to discuss the use of Chinese medicine in SARS treatment. The chief speaker was Professor Liu Bau-yan, Vice President of the Research Institute of Chinese Medicine. In his deliberation, Liu claimed that herbal preparations were found to be effective for the control of fever in SARS patients; lessening lung fibrosis, and in turn a decrease of the mortality rate. The preparations described were found to be equivalent to those described in the previous paragraphs.[9]

Liu then described at length, the results of the only multiple-center control trial, on the use of herbal medicine for SARS treatment. The end points of the control study included: relief of symptoms, shortening of disease course and lowering of mortality. Six hundred cases were involved and the study lasted for 14 days. Out of the 524 cases with complete records, 204 were treated using modern medicine alone (group A), while 318 received both modern and Chinese medicine (group B). 30% of the cases were considered as severe infections and 70% moderate.

A summary of the end results are given as follows:-

	Group A	**Group B**
Mortality	8 cases	none
Fever control	Gradual decline	Fluctuated more
Symptom control	Acceptable	More smooth
Oxygen saturation	Variable	Normal after 3–5 days
Radiograph	Variable	Better and quicker control
Steroid dosage	Fluctuating	Lower amount

The conclusion was: the favorable results encouraged an earlier intervention with herbal preparations.

We are looking forward to a proper written report on this unique experience. At the moment, clarifications were still required for more details of the selection criteria, details of the modern treatment in both groups A and B and their correlations with herbal supplements, etc. Such details were not given in the conference.

HEALTH PROMOTION ACTIVITIES DURING THE SARS OUTBREAK IN THE CHINESE COMMUNITY

Wan Bing was interpreted as a seasonal disease related to changing of the weather, particularly before and during early summer. The Wan Bing philosophy advocates protection against falling ill as the weather turns increasingly warm and becoming unbearable, or when the reverse is true during autumn. Under this traditional belief, every household in the Chinese community, under the care of senior members, would prepare favorable fruits, soups and herbal drinks to "clear" the heat. When one family member starts running a fever, the other members are all given with the same herbal drink.

What are the herbs used?

The influence of the Wan Bing school of thought is so wide and real that simple "anti-fever" formulae and their derivatives have been commonly known and used for decades.

During the SARS outbreak, people in Hong Kong and the mainland used a lot of herbal preparations in an attempt to protect against getting infected.

Some time in late February 2003, when the outbreak around the Pearl Delta was at its peak, citizens and villagers boiled vinegar to generate an acidic steam to fumigate their households. This practice apparently dates back to centuries ago (might be medieval) and whether it did control any viral spread was never proven. Nevertheless, one fringe benefit of this practice must be the increase in awareness within the community of the existence of a contagious disease.

HEALTH PROMOTION ACTIVITIES DURING THE SARS OUTBREAK IN HONG KONG

Although introducing herbal treatment to the hospitals has been an accepted policy of the Hospital Authority in Hong Kong, it was slow to implement so that proper inclusion of herbal therapy as part of the SARS treatment is not ready yet.

A telephone interview was conducted in March 2003 to investigate citizens' attitude towards the use of dietary supplements and herbs as preventive measures against SARS. This survey revealed that only 30–40% of people were actively practicing dietary supplement, using either herbal drinks or vitamins.[10] As more and more people became infected, many Chinese medicine clinics, herbalists and herbal suppliers put forward different herbal preparations for preventive use and business became better and better as the outbreak continued.

One tragic phenomenon of the SARS outbreak was that more and more hospital front-line workers became infected, in spite of enforcement of better of personal protection, during treatment of patients. The Administration tried to help by encouraging academic institutions to consider working on prophylactic herbal preparations. The Chinese University of Hong Kong, has created a herbal formula for prophylactic use by hospital front-line workers on a research trial basis. The research was designed as an observational study on the prophylactic value of a herbal formula against SARS infection among the at risk front-line healthcare workers in the hospitals. The study was initiated by the Hospital Authority of Hong Kong,[1] whose aim was to make sure that each and every front-line worker could be offered the free choice of a preventive option against the contagious disease. A control group was not feasible in this case because the research was launched during the peak of the SARS crisis. The study aimed at providing as many front-line hospital workers as possible with an innovative herbal formula which might have positive effects on the early phases of viral infections affecting the respiratory system. They were advised to take the recommended dose daily for a period of two weeks, at the end of which, they were requested to return a completed questionnaire on adverse

---

[1]The Hospital Authority in Hong Kong is the Employer of all Health Workers working in the Hospitals and Family Clinics.

effects, symptomatology of the influenza, symptoms that the Chinese medicine physician considered as related to Wan Bing, and quality of life (mental health and vitality subscales of SF-36 Questionnaire).

THE HERBAL FORMULA

The herbal formula was created from two herbal formulae in popular use for the prevention and treatment of the early stages of influenza-like syndrome. The first formula Xuang-Ju Yim (XJY) (桑菊飲) has been widely used in southern China and the second, Yu-Ping Fang San (YPFS) (玉屏風散) was popular in central and northern China.[11] Since SARS was a viral infection, a formula that has stronger antiviral effects than XJP and YPFS would be preferred. Two additional herbs known to possess strong antiviral properties in modern herbal pharmacopedia, viz. *Folium Isatidis* (大青葉) and *Scutellaria Boicallensis* (黃芩) were thus added. The new herbal formula was expected to be useful against the early stages of influenza-like viral infections, in other words, useful for the prevention of development of pneumonia. Blood samples were taken from the volunteers who agreed to take the herbal remedy. They were checked for their state of immunological *composition* before, during and after herbal consumption. The herbal preparation was manufactured according to recommendations given by WHO.[12] The herbs were boiled to form a decoction which was subsequently freeze-dried to form pellets for the reconstitution of convenient drinks. The manufacturing line followed the code of practice of good manufacturing practice. Volunteers for the clinical trial were fully informed of the mode of administration; duration of use; possible adverse effects; contraindications; and the contents of the full formula. The results of our preventive regime, using the herbal formula, have been very encouraging. Over 3000 healthcare workers received the herbal preparation, 1100 returned their questionnaires, and 1037 copies were suitable for analysis. During the period that volunteers were being recruited, 69 healthcare workers became infected with SARS. None of these 69 newly infected workers consumed our herbal drink. During this period, 338 healthcare workers were infected, amounting to 0.9% of the total 36,570 workers. This contrast well with the 0% among those who took the herbal drink ($p = 0.006$).

One hundred and twenty-five of the volunteers reported about the different types of adverse symptoms. Table 1 shows the details. None of

Table 1 Adverse Events

Onset of Adverse Symptoms

Day 1:	34	Day 6:	3
Day 2:	41	Day 7:	5
Day 3:	16	Day 10:	1
Day 4:	14	Day 12:	1
Day 5:	9	Day 14:	1

– No. of volunteers reporting : 125/3160
– No. of volunteers who stopped taking after adverse events: 102/3160
– No. of volunteers who continued taking after adverse events: 23/3160

Types of Adverse Symptoms

General		Gastrointestinal		Allergic Response		Musculoskeletal	
Giddiness	34	Epigastric discomfort	32	Rash	5	Tiredness	5
Headache	21	Loose stool	20	Tongue/face swelling	2	Muscleache	2
Feverishness	9	Abdominal discomfort	4			Muscle tightness	2
Chilliness	5						
Sweating	3						
Sore throat	6						
Shortness of breath	1						
Tachycordia	3						
Not sleeping well	1						
Total	83		56		7		9

the adverse effects was serious: 102 stopped taking the herbal preparation, while 23 continued taking it. Using the SF-36 for the assessment of mental health and vitality, it was found that during the two weeks of herb-taking, there were clear improvements in both mental health and vitality. (Figs. 1 & 2). Under the stressful situations of patient care in the epidemic crisis, nurses and healthcare workers tended to experience muscle pain, headache, tiredness and feverishness. In the two weeks of herbal

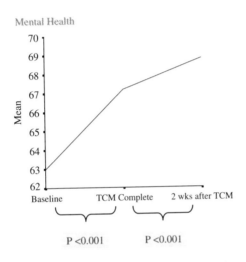

Fig. 1 Change of mental health after herbal consumption.

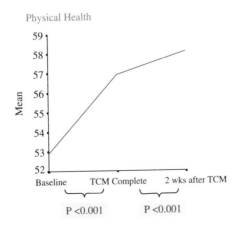

Fig. 2 Change of physical health after herbal consumption.

drink administration, there were noticeable improvements in these symptoms (Figs. 3, 4, 5, 6). Bowel habits and sleep pattern improved during the consumption of the herbs (Figs. 7 & 8) Thirty-seven healthy volunteers were given the oral TCM daily for 14 days. Blood samples were taken on days 0, 15 and 29 for lymphocyte immunophenotyping, complete blood count, differential count, renal and liver function tests, lactic dehydrogenase and creatine kinase analysis. Each volunteer also completed a questionnaire for additional health assessment. Two volunteers

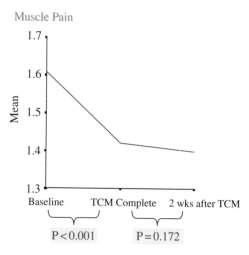

Fig. 3 Symptom of muscle pain after herbal consumption.

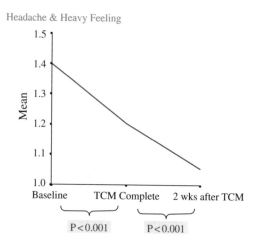

Fig. 4 Symptom of headache after herbal consumption.

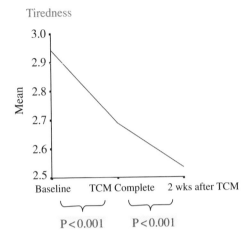

Fig. 5 Feeling of tiredness after herbal consumption.

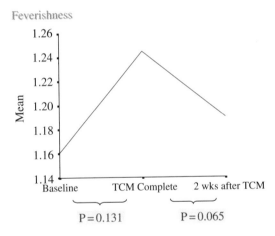

Fig. 6 Feeling of feverishness after herbal consumption.

Fig. 7 Stool condition after herbal consumption.

	Baseline	**TCM Completion**	**2 wks after TCM Completion**
Soft	83%	70.8%	83.1%
Loose	8.1%	23.2%	9.9%
Watery	0.3%	1%	0.4%
Hard	8.6%	5%	6.5%

$$P = 0.025 \qquad P < 0.001$$

Fig. 8 Sleep pattern after herbal consumption.

	Baseline	TCM Completion	2 wks after TCM Completion
Excellent	15%	19%	18%
Quite Good	46%	51%	53%
Not Very Good	35%	28%	27%
Bad	4%	2%	2%

$P < 0.001$ $P = 0.512$

withdrew on day 2 due to headache and dizziness. All the others (18 males, 17 females) remained well with no side effects. No study subject showed any changes in their biochemical tests. There were no derangements in total white cells and lymphocytes, but the CD4/CD8 (helper/suppressor) ratio of T lymphocytes increased significantly from 13.1 ± 0.5 on day 0 to 14.1 ± 0.6 on day 15 ($p = 0.015$), returning to the initial level on day 29. The B-lymphocyte count (cell/μl), however, decreased from 282 ± 142 on day 0 to 263 ± 99 on day 15, and 247 ± 94 on day 29, both $p < 0.05$. There was no gender difference in these changes. Both the transient increase in CD4/CD8 ratio and the persistent decrease in B-lymphocyte should likely be due to the TCM intake. It was concluded that administration of the innovative anti-viral TCM might have beneficial immunomodulatory effects.

Apart from the preventive program, integrated treatment using Chinese herbs and modern medicine was also started later in Hong Kong. As there was a strong request from the local community for the use of herbal medicine in the treatment of SARS infection, two Chinese medicine experts were invited from Guangzhou to participate in the treatment programs. Unlike China, Hong Kong was still deficient of established mechanisms for the proper collaboration between the modern practitioner and the herbalist. The two experts from China, therefore, had a difficult time working out the means of collaboration. It would not be possible to direct research trials of an evidence based nature on behalf of the two experts. The results of treatment, expectedly, would not be comparable to those obtained in China because the integrated treatment was administered in very much a haphazard fashion. Most of the time, integrated treatment was started when patients and their relatives strongly requested for a trial use of a Chinese medicine because the patients were facing obvious survival difficulties.

THE LESSONS WE HAVE LEARNED FROM THE SARS OUTBREAK

An integrated system of Feverish contagious diseases called Wan Bing was founded by two Chinese medicine physicians Yeh Tien-zi and Chen Pin-bo during the early period of the Qing Dynasty. The system was a complete one: from diagnosis, through clinical manifestation, to treatment and prevention.[13]

The course of events in a SARS patient followed quite closely that of the much more familiar influenza, viz., feverishness, fever, malaise, muscle aches, chills, cough, shortness of breath and pneumonia. The main differences lie in the speed of infection and the apparently much higher incidence of pneumonia among the SARS victims.

Wan Bing scholars had different ways of defining the course of events, being based on the severity and behavior of the affected patient. The best established theory could simply be described by four terms: Wai (衛), Qi (氣), Yin (營), Zhur (血), which have been interpreted either as the stages of clinical manifestation or alternatively, the different principles of management at different stages of clinical manifestation. In the former context, Wai and Qi mean early onset of feverishness and running nose; Yin and Zhur mean deterioration of respiratory symptoms ending in hemoptysis. In the latter context of understanding, Wai-Qi is a therapeutic approach whereby the Qi needs to be protected; and later, as the disease progresses, the Zhur component, i.e. the real essence of vitality, is being challenged and hence requires laborious support.

If Chinese medicine works well for Wan Bing, which is related to either influenza or contagious diseases of the respiratory system, one might have little hesitation using herbal remedy during the early stages of influenza, perhaps including SARS, when life support and other specific treatment are yet not required. It is therefore logical to suggest that, Chinese medicine be seriously considered as treatment options during the early stages of viral infections affecting the respiratory tract, but should play only a supportive role when the disease progresses. Modern medications like antibiotics and other more specific items like steroids, should not be given at the early stages, but should be administered only when observations confirmed the seriousness of the disease and their use is clearly indicated. Using Chinese herbal preparations at the observational stages, therefore, would be a logical practical supplement.

Now that the SARS epidemic has subsided, reports from Beijing indicated that about 50% of the SARS patients had received both modern treatment and Chinese herbal adjuvant therapy, and that the use of the herbs had helped speed up the control of fever, and reduce the dosage of steroids.

In June, a German laboratory reported on the *in vitro* effects of an active extract from the herb, liquorice, in the control of SARS-CoV. The report has inspired further study of the various herbs used in Wan Bing.[14]

DISCUSSION

While Chinese communities have, for centuries, been consuming herbal drinks for purposes of prevention or treatment of influenza-like respiratory ailments, none of these drinks have been subjected to proper scientific tests or clinical trials. When Cinatl *et al.* in Germany reported that an extract component of liquorice roots, viz. glycyrrhinzin, had remarkable *in vitro* effects against corona-virus infection, and the quantitative assessment appeared even better than the antiviral pharmaceuticals, there must have been an increase in interests on the research of herbs already known to possess antiviral effects. SARS, as a new viral infection, has threatened the health and well-being of people around the world. It might never appear again or it might return, as an epidemic or hopefully, as an endemic. We are yet uncertain about the possibilities. However, influenza, another viral infection affecting the respiratory tract, for more than one and a half centuries, had threatened men's health and had come and gone many times, killing many people every time it came as an epidemic. While the creation of an effective vaccine would be the most logical solution to the problem of SARS, the difficulties already encountered for AIDS and Influenza, are valuable reminders that science, in the strictly conventional sense, might take time for maturation. Hence, before the day that the viral respiratory infection could be completely brought under control using science, there is a place for the exploration of other means, like herbal alternative medicine, in the treatment, and particularly, in the prevention of frank infection developing into pneumonia.

China has claimed better clinical results of treatment in the fight against the SARS infection. There have been speculations that the lower mortality and morbidity could be due to the use of Chinese medicine. The results from research observations on the prevention of infection using herbs during the SARS crisis did not prove beyond doubts that the herbal formula was effective. Nevertheless, the results did suggest that the formula was safe, it improved the quality of life, and kept those healthcare workers who volunteered were free from the symptoms suggestive of a viral infection, with none of them becoming infected. On the other hand 69 other healthcare workers who did not consume the herbal drink became infected within the same period.

Subsequent research work would be indicated and should include the following areas:

(1) Studies on individual herbs and the mechanism of their antiviral properties;
(2) Studies on individual herbs and the mechanism of their immuno-modulation properties; and perhaps
(3) A wider preventive program in anticipation of another influenza endemic or epidemic in the coming winter.

CONCLUSION

We may be amazed by the interesting results of the trial on the prevention of SARS infection using the herbal preparation. Although no definite conclusion could be made on the scientific efficacy of the herbs, viewing from the perspective of quality of life, the herbal preparation did help. In a Chinese community, a cultural issue like Chinese medicine elicits sentimental reactions. During the SARS outbreak, advocates of the use of Chinese medicine stressed that using Chinese medicine jointly with modern medicine gave much better results. Before objective data become available, one must refrain from being over-optimistic; neither should one make unnecessary premature judgments to the contrary.

REFERENCES

1. Klemman A. Medicine in Chinese culture: Comparative studies of healthcare in China and other countries. US Department of Health,

Education and Welfare, Washington DC, 1975; Centre for Disease Control and Prevention, Ministry of Health, China.

2. Liu C. Looking back at the argument between Chanydia and coronavirus. http://www.satcm.gov.cn/lanmu/feidian/tcm030605hongtao.htm.

3. Instonctions on the treatment of SARS. http://www.satcm.gov.cn/lanmu/feidian/tcm030606jieshao.htm.

4. Zhang Zhon-jung. *Shang-han Luen*, (Chinese Classic).

5. School of Chinese Medicine Chinese University, Curriculum of study: Wan Bing. Faculty of Science Prospectus, 2003, Ministry of Health, China.

6. Treatment of SARS http://www.satcm.gov.cn/lanmu/feidian/030529/liangan.htm.

7. University Grant Council, Hong Kong, Report after a medical team visit to China. University grant council publication, 2001.

8. Media Interview. Control of SARS in Beijing. 30 June 2003, New China Agency.

9. Liu Bo Yan. SARS treatment — the Beijing Experience. SARS conference, polytechnic University, 14 July 2003.

10. Wong E. Survey on the Hong Kong Community for dietary supplements on the prevention of SARS, Clinical Trial Centre for Chinese Medicine, Chinese University of Hong Kong, June 2003.

11. Xuang Ju Yim, Yu Ping Fang Sau. *Chinese Herbal Pharmacopaedia*. Practical Prescriptions in Chinese Medicine. Shenxi Publisher of Science and Technology, 1991.

12. World Health Organisation. General Guide lines for methodologies on Research and Evaluation of Traditional Medicine. WHO, Geneva, 2000.

13. Lin JY, KOHS *Immunology in Chinese Medicine*. Wang Wun Publisher, Taiwan 1993.

14. Cinate J, Morgenstern B, Baner G. Glycyrrhizin, an active component of Liquorice roots and replication of SARS associated corona-virus. *Lancet* **361**(9374): P2045–46,2003.

15. Chan H.Q *et al.* Cancer and Chinese Medicine. http://www.cjmedia.com.cn/ch/article/20030327/20030327073912_1.xml.

16

Long-term Complications of Severe Acute Respiratory Syndrome

Vincent Wong

The mortality of SARS has been reported to range from 6–16%. While the majority of patients recovered from the illness, long term complications of the condition had just started to emerge. The complications of SARS can be divided into those resulting from the disease itself and those resulting from treatment (Table 1). It must be emphasized that since the illness is only described not long ago, the full range of impacts may not be apparent.

DISEASE-SPECIFIC COMPLICATIONS

The lungs are primarily involved in SARS. During active disease, multiple ground glass opacities are present in bilateral lung fields as shown on chest radiographs and computed tomography. The picture resembles bronchiolitis obliterans organizing pneumonia (BOOP). Many disease mechanisms have been proposed. One popular hypothesis is that viral pneumonitis occurs at the beginning, followed by immune-mediated self destruction in the second week of the disease.

Table 1 Complications of Severe Acute Respiratory Syndrome

Complications attributable to SARS activity
    Pulmonary fibrosis
    Respiratory muscle weakness
    Critical illness myopathy / neuropathy
    Depression, anxiety, insomnia

Complications related to steroids
    Adrenal suppression
    Hyperglycemia
    Dyslipidemia
    Cataracts
    Avascular necrosis
    Osteoporosis
    Iatrogenic Cushing's
    Steroid myopathy
    Mood disturbance
    Steroid psychosis
    Superimposed infections

Complications related to ribavirin
    Hemolytic anemia
    Thrombocytopenia, leucopenia, reticulocytosis
    Sleep disturbance, irritability, anxiety, depression
    Arrhythmia

Complications related to Kaletra
    Hyperglycemia
    Dyslipidemia
    Hyperamylasemia

In the acute setting, respiratory failure is common. More than half of the SARS patients required supplementary oxygen, and 20% to 60% required intensive care. The lungs of SARS patients are stiff with fibrosis and difficult to ventilate. Among patients on invasive ventilation, around 35% developed barotraumas. Both pneumothorax and pneumomediastinum have been reported.

With diffuse inflammation, it is possible that permanent damage results. In fact, lung fibrosis is evident as early as one month post-SARS in some patients (Fig. 1). Fortunately, alveolar damage is not prominent in most patients. In Hong Kong, all the patients have full lung function test around two to three months post-SARS. Only five percent had a carbon monoxide diffusion coefficient below 80% of the predicted value.

On the other hand, patients with SARS tend to have a restrictive pattern of lung dysfunction on post-disease testing (defined as forced

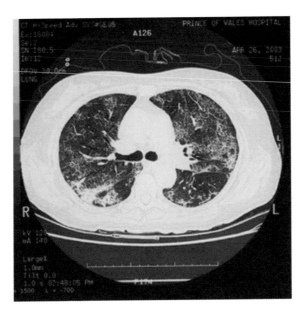

Fig. 1 Computerized tomography of the lung of a 57-year-old SARS patient. Extensive fibrosis was noted just 4 weeks after patient acquired SARS.

expiratory volume in one second over forced vital capacity (FEV_1/FVC above 80%). In most of the cases, lung fibrosis is not extensive enough to explain this picture. Our group subsequently found that the maximal pressure at inspiration and expiration in SARS patients is markedly reduced. Apparently, the restrictive pattern of pulmonary dysfunction is due to neuromuscular weakness. The possible causes of neuromuscular weakness include critical illness myopathy and/or neuropathy, and steroid myopathy.

Mood disorders are also common after SARS. Depression, anxiety and insomnia occur in most patients. We surveyed all patients after they were discharged from hospital. Using the Medical Outcomes Study 36-item Short-Form General Health Survey (SF-36), we noted that patients had markedly reduced vitality, role function and perception of health.

The digestive system is often affected as well. Transaminase levels (ALT and AST) were elevated in 20–50% of patients with SARS. Yet, almost all patients recovered from the illness have normalization of transaminase levels. In the Amoy Gardens outbreak, up to 70% had diarrhea. Most patients with diarrhea had their symptoms resolved within two weeks. There is no long term complication of the gastrointestinal tract reported. SARS-associated coronavirus was isolated in colonic biopsies from some of our patients. Hematological manifestations are common. Lymphopenia, leucopenia, thrombocytopenia, anemia and disseminated intravascular coagulopathy have all been well characterized. Nevertheless, most of these manifestations resolve completely upon follow-up.

COMPLICATIONS RELATED TO THE USE OF CORTICOSTEROIDS

The side effects of corticosteroids are well studied. Many side effects, including hyperglycemia and dyslipidemia, often resolve after the drugs are stopped. Other side effects, however, may be more long-lasting and may result in permanent damage. The side effects depend on the dosage and duration of corticosteroids used. Notably, the dosage of corticosteroids used in different centers differs a lot. In one extreme, a hospital in Hong Kong reported universal use of high dose methylprednisolone since admission. On the other hand, many patients in Canada only received replacement dose of hydrocortisone or none at all.

From our analysis, more than half of the patients who received corticosteroids had adrenal suppression and required low-dose steroid replacement to support adrenal functions. The presentations may be very subtle. Most patients only complain of non-specific malaise, and their hemodynamic status are usually stable.

Loss of bone mass has been reported in patients receiving only one dose of corticosteroids. With prolonged corticosteroid administration, the risk of osteoporosis and future fractures increases. Besides, avascular necrosis is another severe orthopedic complication. Cases of avascular necrosis of both hips had been reported in SARS patients who had received high dose steroid therapy (Fig. 2). This complication is particularly difficult to manage. Revascularization surgery and joint replacement are often required. The limitation in mobility can be tremendous.

Two of our patients developed acute psychosis while on treatment. Magnetic resonant imaging of the brain and lumbar puncture were unrevealing. Presumably, they suffered from steroid psychosis. Apart from psychotic symptoms, depression, anxiety and insomnia are also common as a result of the use of corticosteroids.

COMPLICATIONS RELATED TO THE USE OF ANTI-VIRAL DRUGS

Although the *in vitro* activity of ribavirin against SARS-associated coronavirus is poor, it remains the commonest antiviral drug used to treat SARS. Eighty-eight percent to 100% of patients from different major series received ribavirin. This phenomenon is understandable. Firstly, no alternative antiviral drug has been demonstrated to be more effective in the clinical setting. Secondly, the immunomodulatory action of ribavirin may reduce the lung damage in SARS patients.

We gained most of our experience of ribavirin from chronic hepatitis C patients. However, the dose of ribavirin used in SARS is far greater than that used in chronic hepatitis C. Therefore, side effects are more commonly encountered. On the other hand, the dose of ribavirin used for SARS is lower than that for hemorrhagic fever. Besides, the dose of ribavirin used in different centers differs. For example, most SARS patients in Canada received intravenous ribavirin at 4 g per day, while a common starting dose in Hong Kong was 400 mg eight hourly. This also explains the different side effects profiles among different series.

The most common side effect is hematological. Hemolytic anemia occurred in 49–61% of the patients. On average, the drop in hemoglobin level is around 2 to 3 g/dl. It should be emphasized that ribavirin tends to accumulate in erythrocytes. The intracellular half-life is up to weeks and months. Thus, hemolytic anemia may persist for a long time after cessation of ribavirin. Thrombocytopenia and leucopenia have also been reported, but are rather rare. When intravenous ribavirin is administered, sinus bradycardia is common. Fortunately, hemodynamic instability and dangerous arrhythmia seldom occurs.

Kaletra (lopinavir with ritonavir) is a protease inhibitor for the treatment of acquired immunodeficiency syndrome. It has also been used with some success in SARS. The main side effects are gastrointestinal. Nausea, vomiting and diarrhea often develop. Hyperglycemia and hyperlipidemia are also common side effects. Severe hypertriglyceridemia occurs in some cases, and pancreatitis may result in severe cases. Recent reports suggested that cardiovascular and cerebrovascular complications were not increased with the use of protease inhibitors up to 16 months of follow-up.

CONCLUSION

SARS is associated with numerous intermediate and long-term complications. These complications may arise from the disease itself or its treatment. Further studies are required to introduce more effective treatment with fewer side effects.

REFERENCES (KEY)

1. Lee N, Hui D, Wu A, *et al.* A major outbreak of severe acute respiratory syndrome in Hong Kong. *N Engl J Med* 2003;**348**:1986–1994.

2. Poutanen SM, Low DE, Henry B, *et al.* Identification of severe acute respiratory syndrome in Canada. *N Engl J Med* 2003;**348**:1995–2005.

3. Peiris JSM, Chu CM, Cheng VCC, *et al.* Clinical progression and viral load in a community outbreak of coronavirus-associated SARS pneumonia: A prospective study. *Lancet* 2003;**361**:1767–1772.

4. Booth CM, Matukas LM, Tomlinson GA, *et al.* Clinical features and short-term outcomes of 144 patients with SARS in the Greater Toronto Area. *JAMA* 2003;**289**:2801–2809.

5. Lew TWK, Kwek TK, Tai D, *et al.* Acute respiratory distress syndrome in critically ill patients with severe acute respiratory syndrome. *JAMA* 2003;**290**:374–380.

6. Fowler RA, Lapinsky SE, Hallett D, *et al.* Critically ill patients with severe acute respiratory syndrome. *JAMA* 2003;**290**:367–373.

17

Mental Health Impact of the Severe Acute Respiratory Syndrome Disaster in Hong Kong

Yun Kwok Wing, Chi Ming Leung,
Irene Kam, Sing Lee

INTRODUCTION

The global outbreak of severe acute respiratory syndrome (SARS) has created a disastrous state of chaos and panic across the world. Thought to be originated from southern China, SARS has spread to 32 countries or regions, resulting in 8,437 cases of SARS within a few months of the pandemic.[1] About 20% of them required intensive care admission and a substantial proportion of the patients needed mechanical ventilation.[2,3] Mortality rates of 15–17% have been reported in Hong Kong, Singapore and Canada.[1] The health toll of high morbidity and mortality rate was paralleled by the acute and sudden onset of the outbreak, the highly contagious nature of the disease, the uncertain natural course, and the rapid but unsettled evolution of the understanding of the SARS-CoV virus and treatment.[4–6]

The whole SARS saga has rightly attracted much needed, and often appropriate, attention and concern from all walks of life and sectors, from

**Table 1 Five Levels of Mental
Health Impact of SARS**

1. general population
2. patients
3. patients' families
4. healthcare workers
5. stigma

local government to international health authorities, from medical personnel to lay public.[6] Ostensibly, there is a multitude of impacts of SARS on the various facets of the society. Travel warnings by the World Health organization (WHO) to the affected regions, temporary suspension of schools, significant deleterious effect on the economy, serious disruption to social and family transactions are just a few conspicuous examples. The SARS epidemic has thus created a large-scale disaster with multi-level and far reaching impacts on the community of Hong Kong. Disasters of this scale frequently expose vulnerabilities of the healthcare system and the community infrastructures as they attempt to cope with its adverse impacts.[7] Understandably, SARS has a tremendous effect on the mental health and well being of the society at large, and on individual patients and their families in particular.

The scope of the mental health impact of SARS should at least cover 5 levels (see Table 1). In this chapter, we will briefly discuss the various aspects of the mental health repercussions but with more focus on detailed discussion of the identification and management of the mental health problems of SARS patients.

MENTAL HEALTH IMPACT OF SARS IN THE GENERAL POPULATION

The impact of SARS on the general public can hardly be overemphasized. The shocking news and images of a deadly, previously unknown and highly infectious disease, propagated through intense media coverage, has penetrated every sector and individual citizen. Rising counts of SARS cases and fatalities served to remind us of the vulnerabilities and powerlessness of modern society. However, there is a dearth of data on how the general public mobilizes and utilizes resources in combating SARS or other disasters. In facing the SARS disaster, the general public, like an individual, would have gone through different phases of reaction.[7] The initial shock and denial phase was quickly replaced by the active coping stage at which the resources were drawn together in combating SARS. The anxiety of the community was heightened in coping with the disaster. This was matched by the intense need for personal infection control and appropriate measures for the prevention of SARS on an individual level. Psychological reactions may be aggravated due directly to the SARS disaster (such as threat of SARS, loss of relatives, loss of economic and political stability, reports of the death and sacrifice of medical personnel) as well as to the disruption of the social and family fabric in everyday life. Based on the data from other natural or man-made disasters, various levels of anxiety, insomnia, panic and depression occurred in the acute phase, followed by long-term impacts that could last for years.[7,8] Ongoing studies are aimed at finding out the impact of SARS on the mental well being of Hong Kong citizens. Preliminary data from a random telephone survey of over 800 subjects reported an elevated rate of depression, anxiety, sleep disturbances and post-traumatic stress disorder during the acute phase of SARS.[9] More detailed analysis is being done and the final results will soon be available. The fact that most of these mental health problems are treatable via psychological or/and pharmacological means suggests a parallel need of mental health intervention for the general public.[7] There have been some educational media programs, telephone hotlines and walk-in counseling services for the general public, but systematic evaluation of their effectiveness is required.

It is likely that the experience of disasters may also bring about positive mental health changes, such as increased community cohesiveness, resilience, collective civil action, and changes in spiritual values that can benefit both individuals and the community at large. In order to assess the magnitude of the mental health impact of SARS, including negative and positive aspects, acute and long-term issues, a comprehensive study of the general population is needed.

MENTAL HEALTH IMPACT OF SARS IN PATIENTS' FAMILIES

Once SARS is suspected in a family, the family members and close contacts will be required to be quarantined, restriction is imposed on traveling and their movements will be closely monitored by the health authority.[10] Not only do the family members of SARS patients face the seclusion, isolation, social and occupational disruption, discrimination and stigma, they also need to face other stresses such as fear of cross-infection, grief reaction to injury and loss of family members as well as economic burden.

MENTAL HEALTH IMPACT OF SARS IN HEALTHCARE WORKERS

The outbreak of SARS could be seen as an occupational hazard occurring out of a sudden.[5,6] The huge impact of SARS on healthcare workers and the system can be attributed to its sudden onset, as well as the rapidity of transmission, high rate of infection among healthcare workers and apparently continuing cross-infection despite the increasingly better infection control. The vulnerability of personal safety was compounded by worries about the possibility of cross-infection to family members and friends as well as the duty and responsibility as a healthcare worker.[6] As a result, most of the HCWs adopted either a self-imposed quarantine/isolation or had only minimal family and social interaction. The whole scenario was further complicated by the initial uncertainty of the etiological agent and route of transmission as well as the intense media coverage of the inadequate communication between hospital administrators and frontline workers and the initial shortfall in supply of infection control gears (such as N-95 masks). The whole healthcare community was further shocked by the series of mortalities of healthcare workers who contracted SARS while they were taking care of SARS patients.[11] It is not surprising that HCWs would experience a whole complexity of psychological reactions including fear, frustration, anger, helplessness, isolation, anxiety and depression.[12] The mental health impact on HCWs is understandably huge.

Local hospitals as well as voluntary agencies have provided support and counseling and critical incident debriefing in managing the psychological impact of SARS in healthcare workers, but the effectiveness of such measures remains unclear. Systematic studies in assessing the psychological impact, both negative and positive, on HCWs of all ranks are needed.

STIGMATIZATION OF SARS

Stigmatization and discrimination have been part and parcel of the human history involving infectious diseases such as leprosy and HIV for a long time.[13] The health and economic effects fueled by stigmatization and discrimination are devastating. Expectedly, SARS has not only resulted in physical morbidities, but also generated a series of labeling and stigmatic effects on both SARS patients and their close contacts. While the need for proper protection and isolation of potential carriers of the SARS virus was understandable, there were times that such discrimination and stigmatization was disproportional to the real threat. Stigmatization is one major factor that obstructs help seeking, perpetuates psychiatric morbidity, decreases the willingness of individuals to co-operate with preventative measures, and jeopardizes public health interventions.

The twin effect of stigmatization and discrimination was also evident in Toronto, where there was a major outbreak of SARS outside Asia. As SARS was thought to have originated and been imported from southern China, Asian communities and even Asian patients reported considerable stigmatization and racist reactions.[12] In Hong Kong, from the end of March to July 28, 2003, the Equal Opportunities Commission of Hong Kong (EOC) received more than 520 enquiries and complaints from the public as a result of possible discrimination related to SARS. A telephone survey on SARS-related interpersonal difficulties was conducted by the EOC and Hong Kong Mood Disorders Centre (HMDC) of the Department of Psychiatry, The Chinese University of Hong Kong, from 3 July to 8 July, 2003. One thousand and twenty-three randomly selected respondents aged 15 to 64 (491 males and 532 females; 591 employees, 132 students and 167 housewives) were interviewed.[14] The findings of the survey showed that over 70% of the respondents were anxious about contracting SARS, and half of them believed that people would still be scared of individuals who had already recovered from SARS. Most respondents attributed anxiety about SARS to: (a) inadequate information from the government as well as its slow response and poor coordination (over 70%); (b) frequently changing information from medical professionals (nearly 70%); and (c) strong emphasis on morbidity and mortality rate in the mass media (over 40%).

At the peak of the SARS outbreak in April 2003, 65%, 50% and 31% respectively of the respondents, who were employed, would tend to avoid their colleagues who: (a) had a fever; (b) resided in buildings where SARS cases were found; and (c) had family members who had contracted SARS. By July 2003, 16% would avoid colleagues who had recovered from SARS in the workplace. In both April and July, respondents would prefer employers to take preventive measures against workers considered to be at increased risk of contracting SARS. In schools, 11% of the student respondents would distance themselves from classmates who had recovered from SARS. As regards the seeking of employment, 21% of the respondents perceived that employers would mind taking job applicants if the latter or their family members were previously infected with SARS, and if they resided in previously high-risk buildings. Given two applicants with identical educational background, experience and competence but one of them had recovered from SARS, 49% of the respondents perceived that employers would prefer the non-SARS applicant. These findings indicated that negative attitudes and practices towards people previously affected by or connected with SARS could remain even after their recovery. Continued intersectoral efforts on education, channels for handling complaints, and comprehensive guidelines for employers and employees will help reduce discrimination.

MENTAL HEALTH IMPACT IN SARS PATIENTS

The mental health impact in SARS patients can be divided into acute, early recovery, short and longer-term phases. During the acute phases, the patients were admitted to hospital for about 3 weeks' treatment once they were suspected or confirmed of having SARS.[2,3,15–17] A standard protocol for the acute treatment of SARS in Hong Kong has been adopted by most of the centers.[2,16–17] However, the medical treatment of SARS remains controversial and requires further refinement.[6,17] Briefly, a combination of antiviral agent, ribavirin and corticosteroid (including oral, parenteral and pulse therapy) was employed, in addition to the general supportive measures, oxygen therapy and assisted ventilation in a high percentage of patients.[2–3,16–17]

The course of illness of SARS was variable and range from relatively mild symptoms of fever, cough and malaise to a severe debilitating disease with acute respiratory distress syndrome requiring intensive care and mechanical ventilation and fatalities.[2–3,6,17] Ostensibly, SARS patients needed to face a multitude of stress and problems (Tables 2 and 3). Because of the potential of cross-infection, the hospitalization of SARS patients also served as a quarantine measure. Throughout the hospital stay, a no-visitor policy was strictly implemented. Understandably,

**Table 2 Potential Etiologies of
Psychiatric Morbidities
of SARS Illness — Five S**

1. Seclusion and alienation
2. Sleep and sensory deprivation
3. SARS illness
4. Steroid and ribavirin
5. Stigmatization

**Table 3 Common Stressors during SARS Illness across
Different Phases of Illness**

Acute Phase:
1. Quarantine measures with no-visitor policy: Seclusion, alienation, boredom
2. Elicitation of horror, worries, fear, uncertainty and helplessness
3. Witness of deterioration of others and self
4. Family co-infection
5. Sleep disruption and sensory deprivation
6. Physical debilitation: Fever, malaise, pain
7. SARS Co-V: Currently no concrete evidence of CNS involvement
8. Treatment: Neuropsychiatric side effect of steroid and possibly ribavirin
9. Course of illness: Hypoxemia, ICU admission and ventilation
10. Treatment environment: Cared by HCW highly "armed" with infection-control gears with possible more distant therapist-patients relationship

Early Recovery Phase:
1. Physical debilitation: General, pulmonary, endocrine, muscular and neuropsychiatric
2. Worries about cross-infection to others and re-infection
3. Discrimination and stigmatization
4. Family and social rejection
5. Grief: Death of family members due to SARS
6. Economic and occupational problems

Medium and Long-term Phase:
1. Physical debilitation
2. Stigmatization
3. Grief
4. Worry over re-infection
5. Economic and occupational problems

feeling of alienation and loneliness among SARS patients were not uncommon. The feeling of alienation was further accentuated by the need of careful infection control and apparently more distant therapist-patient encounters. The uncertainty and unpredictability of the course of the SARS illness, the highly infectious nature of the disease, co-infection within the families, the need to care for the rest of the unaffected family members, were some common worries and burden of SARS patients. For those patients who have a relatively milder illness, prolonged hospitalization meant the lack of routine engagement and feeling of boredom. In the face of this series of stresses, a series of psychopathologies and psychiatric morbidities were seen in patients. A complex emotional reaction involving worries, fear, angry and helplessness was common during this acute phase.[12] We reported the initial series of SARS patients who were referred for further psychiatric evaluation in the Prince of Wales hospital.

PSYCHIATRIC CONSULTATION DURING THE INITIAL ACUTE PHASE

During the initial one-month that followed the outbreak of SARS on 8 March 2003, six SARS patients (3 men and 3 women, mean age = 36) out of a total of 138 SARS cases (referral rate 4.3%) who were registered during the period, were referred for psychiatric evaluation. All psychiatric diagnoses were made according to DSM-IV.[18] All contracted the disease in the first wave of the infection and fulfilled the criteria for SARS proposed by the WHO case definition.[19] All received ribavirin and high dose steroid, with a mean dose of 179 mg prednisolone equivalent daily for 12 days. Four required ICU care and one, mechanical ventilation. Four patients with mental disorders (two with mania and two with delirium) due to general medical condition/substance induced (GMC/SI) and two with prominent adjustment disorder with mixed anxiety and depressive features, were diagnosed. The patients with mental disorders due to GMC/SI had negative CT brain findings, three of whom also had normal MRI brain findings. While the other one showed mild non-specific EEG changes. The patients with organic mania had onset about two weeks after starting steroid/ribavirin and responded well to olanzapine. The two patients with delirious state had moderate to severe oxygen desaturation, and responded significantly to psychopharmacological intervention when their respiratory status improved. The two subjects with prominent adjustment disorder responded well to psychosocial intervention with occasional hypnotics and anxiolytic. No patients had past psychiatric or family history of mental illness. This initial series of patients illustrated the spectrum of psychiatric morbidities seen in SARS. Especially evident was the predominance of neuropsychiatric complications. The exact etiologies for two cases of organic mania were unclear but the use of high dose steroid may be a contributing factor.[20,21] Nevertheless, more detailed analysis with a larger series of patients may shed light on the definitive role of steroid in the SARS-related mood disturbances. The occurrence of delirium highlighted the complex and multi-factorial etiology of organic brain syndromes in SARS patients. A combination of hypoxia, sepsis, co-existing physical illness, isolation with sleep and sensory deprivation, and neurotoxic drugs may all have contributed.[18] The SARS-CoV virus belongs to the coronavirus families and some of them have demyelination effect in animals.[4] Nevertheless, there was no evidence of CNS involvement of SARS-CoV but further investigations are needed to exclude their neurotropic effect. Thus, efforts should be targeted at early identification and treatment as organic mental disorders in SARS subjects undermine prognosis, disrupt strict quarantine procedures, and jeopardize morale among professionals.[22]

Despite the complexity of the conditions and multiple stresses (Tables 2 and 3), only 4.3% of SARS cases with prominent psychiatric morbidities were identified in this study. As the current practice did not have routine psychiatric screening by liaison psychiatrists, it is likely that only the severe and disturbing cases were referred. Mild steroid-induced euphoria might not be detected. Malignant anxiety, guilt and worries could be brushed aside as normal reactions. Masks worn on a manifestly tense ward and fear of cross infection would further deter communication and detection. The low referral rate thus must represent a much under-estimated morbidity.

SYSTEMIC SCREENING OF PSYCHIATRIC MORBIDITIES AMONG SARS PATIENTS DURING EARLY RECOVERY PHASE

In view of the above study and the likelihood of underestimation of psychiatric morbidities among SARS patients, we have started systematic psychiatric screening among all SARS patients at 2–4 weeks after discharge prospectively at the follow-up clinic. All SARS patients who have recovered from the acute illness would usually have a short stay in a rehabilitation facility before discharge back to home. All the SARS patients would then be followed up in the SARS clinic until their physical condition has finally settled. The aim of this study was to determine the prevalence of psychological morbidity and identify those factors associated with increased risk of psychological morbidity in our SARS patients. All the patients were assessed with a semi-structured clinical interview and a battery of psychometric assessments for detection of the psychiatric morbidity and psychosocial functioning. Preliminary data suggested a much higher rate of psychiatric morbidities with more extensive psychopathologies and a full range of psychiatric disorders. Those patients who were found to have significant psychiatric morbidities were referred for further psychiatric treatment in a specialized SARS-psychiatric clinic.

SPECIALIZED SARS-PSYCHIATRIC CLINIC

During the early phase of the clinic, we encountered the problems and concern of potential cross-infection to other psychiatric patients should the clinic be situated in the same physical site of the usual psychiatric clinic.[23] The other major problem was the unwillingness of some of the patients to come for psychiatric or psychological treatment. Some worried about the issue of double stigmatization (stigmatization due to SARS and SARS-related psychiatric morbidities), while others had denial of their psychosocial problems. A specialized SARS Psychiatric Clinic was set up alongside the SARS Follow-up Clinic.

In this cohort clinic, up to the time of writing of the chapter, we have managed 23 SARS patients (20 female and 3 male, mean age = 38.3 years/range (24–67)). 60.8% of them were healthcare workers, the majority of whom were nurses. A whole spectrum of psychiatric morbidity was seen and 34.7% of them had co-morbidity of more than one psychiatric diagnosis (Table 4). The Global Assessment of Functioning of the group had a mean score of 59.7 (SD 12.6).[18] The mean scores of General Health Questionnaire-30 and Beck Depression Inventory were 19.7 (SD 8.6) and 12.4 (SD 7.7), respectively.[24–25] The mean score of Hospital Anxiety and Depression scale was 20.3 (SD 9.4).[26] In other words, the whole group of patients had at least a moderate degree of clinical severity. Over 40% of them were suffering from a major depressive illness which was followed

Table 4 List of Psychiatric Diagnosis among the Patients seen in SARS-psychiatric Clinic

Diagnosis*	Frequency (N)	Percentage (%)
Major depression	12	38.7
PTSD	7	22.6
Adjustment reaction	3	9.7
Psychotic or delirious disorder	2	6.5
Mania or mixed mood disorder	2	6.5
Grief reaction	2	6.5
Acute stress disorder	1	3.2
Panic disorder	1	3.2
Chronic insomnia	1	3.2

*Patients had co-morbid diagnoses.

by post-traumatic stress disorder as the second commonest disorder. A number of them harbored the psychotic, mood and suicidal features without being known and detected by the clinicians.

After consultation in the clinic, 74% of the patients received psychotropic drugs. The commonest group of drugs prescribed was anxiolytics (52.7%), followed by antidepressants (47.8%), hypnotics (34.7%) and major tranquillizers (13%). The successful use of newer atypical antipsychotics in our cases supported the role of using these newer agents in organic mania and psychosis in addition to their role in acute mania.[27] While the possibility of steroid and ribarivin effects could not be ruled out in those patients with depression and PTSD, their similar clinical features and the presence of multiple etiologies will suggest the need to manage them in the same way as for similar conditions in general patients.[28–30]

Use of non-pharmacological intervention is also common. Advice on sleep hygiene, targeted sleep behavioral therapy like stimulus control and sleep restriction therapy was given.[31] Grief counselling for the patients with bereavement was also started. In those patients with depression and PTSD, supportive and cognitive therapy was employed. Two patients were also referred to clinical psychology colleagues for further intensive psychological treatment for their prominent PTSD.[29]

Our experience with SARS patients was consistent with studies on victims of other severe disasters and major illnesses in that there was an increased prevalence of depression, post-traumatic stress disorder and

**Table 5 Psychopharmacological Treatments for
SARS-related Psychiatric Morbidities**

1. Sleep disruption and insomnia: lorazepam, zoplicone, zoplidem
2. Delirium, psychotic and manic state: olanzapine, haloperidol, sulpiride
3. Anxiety: bromazepam, lorazepam, diazepam, alprazolam
4. Depression: sertraline, paroxetine, fluoxetine, mirtazapine, dothiepin
5. Post-traumatic Stress disorder: SSRI, mirtazapine.

**Table 6 Non-pharmacological Treatments for
SARS-related Psychiatric Morbidities**

1. Encouragement of social and family support and reintegration.
2. Sleep hygiene and behavioral therapy (sleep restriction and stimulus control therapy)
3. Supportive psychotherapy
4. Cognitive-behavioral psychotherapy (CBT) for depression and anxiety
5. Special behavioral and cognitive therapy for PTSD eg. CBT, Eye movement desensitization therapy.

suicide rates.[2,3] We believe that routine screening, heightened awareness, timely consultation, appropriate medical and social intervention would be the key elements in tackling the SARS-related psychiatric morbidities. The favorable responses by most of the patients supported the need for earlier identification and treatment.

REMEDIAL SUGGESTIONS FOR PREVENTING AND MANAGING THE PSYCHIATRIC AND PSYCHOSOCIAL MORBIDITIES RELATED TO SARS

There has been warning that SARS may return in the coming winter. While optimism in dealing with another SARS outbreak is supported by the rapid scientific advances, more attention should also be paid to the management and prevention of the psychosocial consequences of SARS (Table 7).

Acute Phase

1. Avoidance of alienation. One of the main problems of SARS patients who are admitted to hospitals is their complex psychological

**Table 7 Remedial Suggestions for Preventing and Managing
the Associated Stressors related to SARS**

Acute Phase:
1. Use of modern technology like mobile phones, video-conference, internet facilities to enhance the social and familial support and communication may help to achieve the effect of isolation but not alienation
2. Sleep hygiene and p.r.n. hypnotics to promote adequate sleep
3. Adequate symptom control to tackle physical debilitation
4. Newer, safer more target-specific treatment regime
5. More sensitive and routine screening of concealed psychiatric problems during hospital stay especially during ICU admission
6. More homely and friendly treatment environment
7. Early identification of at-risk patients and early psychosocial/psychiatric support and treatment
8. Need for psychiatric-SARS beds or unit for psychotic, manic and suicidal patients

Early Recovery Phase:
1. Rehabilitation programmes to minimize physical debilitation
2. Effective treatment and methods in shortening the virus-shedding period to minimize cross-infection
3. Mass education and society support to tackle discrimination and stigma
4. Enhance social and family support via education, social intervention and network (both governmental and voluntary agencies)
5. Grief counseling
6. Integrated and early psychiatric and psychological intervention for at-risk patients
7. Self-help group

reactions with feeling of alienation, loneliness, boredom, worries and fear. The necessary quarantine with a no-visitor policy further contributed to the perceived lack of familial and social support. In the newly modified infectious wards or hospitals, they should all be equipped with modern electronic communication systems such as mobile phones, video-conference and Internet facilities in order to enhance the social and familial support.

2. Shortening of hospital stay: The rapid understanding of the SARS virus and their immunological consequences should aim to provide more target-specific treatment with shorter hospital stay.

3. Early identification and management of psychological problems: There should be routine screening for any hidden psychosocial morbidities and early identification of at-risk patients (such as those in

ICU patients). An ongoing study is examining the validity of using an easily available self-report questionnaire such as the hospital anxiety and depression scales (HADS) as the screening tool for any hidden psychiatric morbidity. Early psychosocial support and treatment in the form of counseling, drugs and environmental manipulation will be essential. Judicious and brief use of hypnotics and anxiolytics with appropriate sleep hygiene will be of much help in those with sleep disturbances. The role of liaison psychiatrists should be more proactive and be considered as part of the multidisciplinary team in the management of SARS.

4. Need for specialized SARS-psychiatric care: As discussed above, a proportion of SARS patients may develop psychotic, delirious, manic, suicidal and disturbing behavior. The potential and greatly enhanced risk of cross-infection during the control of these SARS patients with unstable mental state is an important issue. The medical staff should have mental health training, adequate protection and close liaison with the psychiatric team.

Recovery Phase

1. Early identification of psychiatric problems: The occurrence of suicide attempts during the early recovery phase illustrated the importance of continuing vigilance during the rehabilitation phase. The close and systemic screening for any hidden psychiatric morbidities is much needed. Grief counseling and support should be implemented for vulnerable subjects.

2. Avoidance of stigmatization: Mass education campaign and mobilization of the resources of the society has already made a strong and positive impact on the society. More attention is needed to destigmatize SARS and their aftermath.

3. Enhance family and social support via education, social intervention and network.

4. SARS-psychiatric clinic: Given the considerable psychiatric morbidities among SARS patients, there is a need for establishing a specialized SARS-psychiatric clinic with experienced personnel.

5. Self-help group: Self-help group may assist their recovery, sharing of the burden and mobilization of resources.

CONCLUSION

The global pandemic of SARS has a great and far-reaching impact on various facets of societies. The effects of SARS on various mental health issues have just started to emerge. Preliminary data suggested that the scale of the mental health impact of SARS has extended beyond the patients and their families, healthcare workers and hospitals to the wider community. Apart from the need for further advances in the understanding of the SARS-CoV virus and the physical management aspects, the healthcare planners, administrators and frontline clinicians should all be equipped with the knowledge and skill in preventing and coping with the mental health impact of SARS, in both the acute phase and in the long-term. Early and accurate identification and treatment of the vulnerable patients would ameliorate psychosocial problems, minimize psychiatric morbidities and facilitate the full rehabilitation of the SARS patients.

REFERENCES

1. WHO data. Cumulative number of reported cases (SARS) from 1 November 2002 to 11 July 2003. *World Health Organization* http://www.who.int/csr/sars/country/2003_07_11/en/.

2. Lee N, Hui D, Wu A, *et al.* A major outbreak of severe acute respiratory syndrome in Hong Kong. *NEJM* 2003;**48**(20):1986–94.

3. Booth CM, Matukas LM, Tomlinson GA, *et al.* Clinical features and short-term outcomes of 144 patients with SARS in the greater Toronto area. *JAMA* 2003;**289**(21):2801–9.

4. Holmes KV. SARS coronavirus: A new challenge for prevention and therapy. *J Clin Invest* 2003;**111**(11):1605–9.

5. SARS: What have we learned. *Nature* 2003;**424**:121–126.

6. Masur H, Emanuel W, Lane HC. Severe Acute Respiratory Syndrome. Providing care in the face of uncertainty. *JAMA* 2003;**289**:2861–2863.

7. Burkle FM. Acute-phase mental health consequences of disasters: Implications for triage and emergency services. *Ann Emerg Med* 1996:119–128.

8. Etienne KG, Marcie-Jo K, John PP, *et al.* Suicide after natural disasters. *NEJM* 1998:373–378.

9. Lau JTF, Tsui HY, Wing YK, Pang E. Psychological Impacts of SARS on the general public in Hong Kong. Presented in the mental health symposium organized by Mental health association of Hong Kong and Hospital Authority on 18 August 2003.

10. Donnelly CA, Ghani AC, Leung GM, *et al.* Epidemiological determinants of spread of causal agent of severe acute respiratory syndrome in Hong Kong. [erratum appears in *Lancet*. 2003;**361**(9371):1832]. *Lancet* 2003;**361**(9371):1761–6.

11. *Ming Pao* Newspaper. Death of the daughter of Hong Kong, late Dr. Tse YM. 22 May 2003.

12. Maunder R, Hunter J, Vincent L, *et al.* The immediate psychological and occupational impact of the 2003 SARS outbreak in a teaching hospital. *CMAJ* 2003;**168**(10):1245–51.

13. Heatherton TF, Kleck RE, Hebel MR, Hull JG (eds). *The Social Psychology of Stigma.* The Guilford Press, New York, 2000.

14. Hong Kong Mood Disorders Center, Department of Psychiatry, The Chinese University of Hong Kong. SARS related difficulties in work and social lives in Hong Kong. (www.hmdc.med.cuhk.edu.hk).

15. Ho W. Hong Kong Hospital Authority Working Group on SARS, Central Committee of Infection Control. Guidelines on management of severe acute respiratory syndrome (SARS). *Lancet.* 2003;**361**(9366): 1313–5.

16. So LK, Lau AC, Yam LY, *et al.* Development of a standard treatment protocol for severe acute respiratory syndrome. *Lancet.* 2003; **361**(9369):1615–7.

17. Wong GW, Hui DS. Severe acute respiratory syndrome (SARS): Epidemiology, diagnosis and management. *Thorax.* 2003; **58**(7):558–60.

18. American Psychiatric Association. Diagnostic and statistical manual of mental disorders. 4th ed. American Psychiatric Association, Washington, 1994.

19. World Health Organization. Case definitions for surveillance of severe acute respiratory syndrome (SARS). www.who.int/csr/sars/ casedefinition/en/.

20. Naber D, Sand P, Heigl B. Psychopathological and neuropsychological effects of 8-days' corticosteroid treatment: A prospective study. *Psychoneuroendocrinology* 1996;**21**:25–31.

21. Boston Collaborative Drug Surveillance Program. Acute adverse reactions to prednisone in relation to dosage. *Clin Pharmacol Ther* 1972;**13**:694–8.

22. McCusker J, Cole M, Abrahamowicz M, *et al.* Delirium predicts 12-month mortality. *Arch Intern Med* 2002;**162**:457–63.

23. Peiris JS, Chu CM, Cheng VC, *et al.* Clinical progression and viral load in a community outbreak of coronavirus-associated SARS pneumonia: A prospective study. *Lancet* 2003;**361**(9371):1767–72.

24. Chan DW, Chan TF. Reliability, validity and the structure of the general health questionnaire in a Chinese context. *Psychol Med* 1983; **13**:363–371.

25. Shek DT. Reliability and factorial structure of the Chinese version of the Beck Depression Inventory. *J Clin Psychol* 1990;**46**(1):35–43.

26. Leung CM, Wing YK, Kwong PK, A Lo, Shum K. Validation of the Chinese-Cantonese version of the Hospital Anxiety and Depression Scale and comparison with the Hamilton Rating Scale of depression. *Acta Psychiatr Scand* 1999;**100**:456–461.

27. Tohen M, Baker RW, Altshuler LL, *et al.* Olanzapine versus divalproex in the treatment of acute mania. *Am J Psychiatry* 2002;**159**(6):1011–7.

28. Wing YK. Recent advances in the management of depression and psychopharmacology. *Hong Kong Med J* 2000;**6**:85–92.

29. Beliles K, Stoudemire A. Psychopharmacologic treatment of depression in the medically ill. *Psychosomatics.* 1998;**39**(3):S2–19.

30. Brunello N, Davidson JR, Deahl M, *et al.* Posttraumatic stress disorder: Diagnosis and epidemiology, comorbidity and social consequences, biology and treatment. *Neuropsychobiology.* 2001;**43**(3):150–62.

31. Lavie P. Sleep disturbances in the wake of traumatic events. *NEJM* 2001;**345**(25):1825–32.

18

Infection Control of SARS in the Hospital

Peter Tong, D Lyon, SF Liu

Severe acute respiratory syndrome (SARS), a newly emerging infectious disease, highlights the importance of infection control measures in containing the spread of a contagious disease. The lack of knowledge on the epidemiology and pathogenesis of SARS renders the implementation of specific preventive measures rather difficult, at least in the earliest phase of the epidemic. SARS behaves mostly as a nosocomial infection, characterized by high levels of transmission among healthcare workers in hospitals. Hospital-related exposure can be identified in more than 22% of cases.[1] The absence of specific treatment or vaccines forces healthcare officials to rely on the empirical processes of isolation and quarantine.[2] Initial efforts to control SARS included isolation of suspect and probable SARS patients, quarantine of contacts of known SARS patients, and use of personal protective equipment (PPE) for healthcare workers and visitors.

Despite these measures, a number of transmission events had occurred even after the index cases had been isolated. Patients with overt symptoms suggestive of SARS were not likely to be responsible for the outbreaks in hospitals, for they were soon kept in isolation with all appropriate measures taken. Rather, patients who were not identified as SARS,

226

and hence not isolated initially, have been responsible for most outbreaks. Unrecognized cases of SARS had led to large-scale infection among hospital staff and subsequent transmission to the community. These super spreading events were seen in different locations, including Hong Kong,[3] Toronto[4] and Taiwan.[5] The absence of specific symptoms and a reliable point-of-care diagnostic test for use in the early phase of the disease calls for vigilance among front-line clinical staff in dealing with patients presenting with upper respiratory illness.

SARS-CoV is transmitted primarily by droplet spread and direct contact. In addition, the outbreak in a residential complex in Hong Kong has been attributed to a fecal route of transmission.[6] Among healthcare workers, cross-infection appears to have occurred following close contact with SARS patients. In implementing appropriate infection control measures for SARS, there are three important aspects to be considered.

ENVIRONMENT

In the era of the widespread practice of vaccination and the availability of powerful antimicrobial agents, infectious diseases have been relegated to a less important agenda in the modern design of hospital wards. The rapid surge in the number of SARS patients has highlighted the lack of isolation facilities in regional hospitals in Hong Kong. More importantly, the hospital ward is not designed to look after highly infectious patients. The lack of negative pressure rooms and single rooms with their own bathroom facilities, the communal washroom, and the open-plan patient areas makes implementation of effective infection control measures difficult.

MODE OF TRANSMISSION

A major mode of transmission of SARS-CoV is through close contact with an infected person, especially following exposure to respiratory or bodily secretions from an infected person. The initial outbreak among healthcare workers at the Prince of Wales hospital has been attributed to the generation of infective fine aerosol droplets from an unidentified SARS patient following the use of a nebulizer.[7] Consequently, precautions are introduced to protect the healthcare workers during aerosol-generating procedures. These measures include the use of PPE and safe-work practices in an airborne isolation environment.

Table 1 Stability of the SARS-Cov in the Hospital Environment (adopted from the WHO report on the stability and resistance of SARS coronavirus compiled by members of WHO laboratory network, accessed 4 May 2003)

	Saline (hours)	Stool (hours)
Plastered wall	24	36
Plastic surface	36	72
Formica surface	36	36
Stainless steel	36	72
Wood	12	24
Cotton cloth	12	24
Glass slide	72	96
Paper file cover	24	36

Cohort placement of SARS patients has been recommended, though not without its own problem. Viral shedding from SARS patients facilitates the spread of the infection by direct contact. Surfaces that are touched frequently (e.g. table tops, door knobs, bed rails and lavatory surfaces) may serve as important media of SARS-CoV transmission. Investigations from member laboratories of the WHO multi-center collaborative network on SARS diagnosis indicate that SAR-CoV can survive up to 36 and 72 hours on solid surfaces and stool, respectively (Table 1). In particular, the virus is stable up to 4 days in stool from patients with diarrhea, who have higher pH than normal stool.[8] Reassuringly, the SARS-CoV loses infectivity following exposure to commonly used cleansing agents such as hypochlorite solution. Hence, cleaning and disinfection of the environmental surfaces constitute an essential part of the infection control measures. The practice of hand washing and glove changing will further reduce the transmission of SARS-CoV by fomites. The importance of hand washing cannot be over-stated. Case-control studies on the effectiveness of measures in preventing noscosmial transmission clearly demonstrated the usefulness of careful hand hygiene.[9]

IMPLEMENTATION OF INFECTION CONTROL POLICY

The availability of potent and broad-spectrum antimicrobial and antiviral agents has lowered healthcare workers' perception of the importance of good infection control practice. With the emergence of SARS, the surge of numerous guidelines on various aspects of infection control highlights the lack of education, training and compliance among healthcare workers of all levels. It is, therefore, imperative that all staff have regular training sessions and practice. The infection control team of the hospital has the main responsibility to draw up and continually review protocols in the light of new information. Designated team members should disseminate the information to all relevant staff. The guidelines should be posted on appropriate settings to improve compliance. To ensure compliance of infection control policies in the hospital or clinic settings, dedicated persons should be appointed to monitor the practice of hospital or clinic staff.

To contain the spread of SARS in hospital, early identification and prompt isolation of suspect or probable cases are essential. Based on our understanding of the disease, the following infection control measures should be included.

1. Screening and Triage

To date, most of the outbreaks of SARS in hospitals are caused by "invisible" or unidentified infected persons. Early identification of suspected or probable SARS patients with appropriate isolation is therefore essential to prevent outbreaks. Upon arrival at the emergency room, all the patients should be advised to wear surgical masks. All the staff must take full precautions against droplet contact and airborne transmission while dealing with patients. Healthcare workers in appropriate protective gears should ask specific questions on fever, respiratory symptoms, recent travel and close contact with a SARS patient before performing other history-taking or examinations. Body temperature should be taken. If fever is present and the SARS screening questions are negative, the patient should be admitted to an infection triage ward where further investigation of the source of pyrexia will be taken (Fig. 1). If the SARS screening is positive, patients should be placed in a SARS triage ward where confirmatory tests will be carried out. Once SARS is confirmed, the patient will be placed in a SARS ward for further observation and management. Patients with suspected or probable SARS should be admitted to a negative pressure room. When negative pressure rooms are not available, patients should be placed in single rooms with their own bathroom facilities. Failing that, they should be cohorted and placed in an area with an independent air circulation system as well as bathroom facilities. All staff dealing with

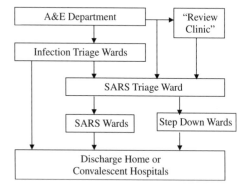

Fig. 1 Algorithm for screening patients at the first point of contact.

SARS patients must practice barrier nursing, using precautions for airborne, droplet and contact transmission. The unit is only open to patients with suspected or probable SARS to avoid cross-infection.[10] For those whose tests do not confirm the presence of SARS, they should be placed in a step-down ward where they will be observed for seven days before they are discharged. Following discharge from the hospital, the patients should continue to practice strict infection control measures. At the Prince of Wales Hospital, a review clinic has been established to monitor ambulatory patients whose signs and symptoms are equivocal for SARS. These patients will be monitored closely with chest radiographs and complete blood count.

Visitors should only be allowed under exceptional circumstances and they should be supervised and required to wear full PPE. Only experienced staff should be deployed in clinical areas where SARS patients are accommodated. Frequent rotation of different staff members should be avoided. All non-essential staff, including students, should not be allowed in the ward.

2. Measures for Ambulatory SARS Patients

Following discharge from the hospital, patients should continue to practice good personal hygiene and infection control measures for 14 days at home. They should limit interactions outside the home and should not report to work or school. Surgical mask should be used. Frequent hand washing is essential, in particular after contact with nose, mouth or respiratory secretions or after going to the toilet. Sharing of food, utensils, towels and bedding with other family members should be avoided. Environmental surfaces should be cleaned daily with diluted household bleach (1 in 100 dilution). In Hong Kong, all SARS patients have to report to designated medical clinics operated by the Department of Health for 10 days following their discharge from hospital.

3. Protection against Droplet, Contact and Airborne Transmission

All persons coming into contact with SARS patients must practice precautions according to the risk of exposure. In general, healthcare settings should be stratified according to the patient- or procedure-related activities into high- and low-risk areas. High-risk patient areas include SARS cohort and screening wards, fever triage areas, intensive care units and specific areas designated for SARS patients. Other patient areas in the hospital are regarded as low-risk zones. The hospital infection control unit should establish the appropriate level of precaution and PPE for each category.[11]

In the high-risk areas, all the staff including ancillary personnel must wear gowns, gloves and eye protective gear (goggles, face-shields or visors), and wash their hands frequently after contact with patients or their environment. Airborne precautions include an isolated room with negative pressure and the use of N95 respirators or respirators of higher specifications (P100 or P99 filters). Ideally, a qualitative fit test should be done for respirators. Gowns, gloves and eye protective gear are indicated for procedures that involve exposure to blood, body fluids, respiratory secretions and excreta (Table 2). Disposable items should not be reused. If N95 respirators are not available, then surgical masks should be worn. In the low-risk areas, surgical masks should be worn by all the staff.

At the peak of the outbreak at the Prince of Wales Hospital, there were concerns about the effectiveness of the water-repellent gowns. Hence, protective suit that is originally designed for chemical spill (Barrier Man®) was used by the healthcare workers on a trial basis. The rationale for the use of Barrier Man was based on the assumption that it would provide better cover for the exposed areas such as the head and neck. However, the lack of ventilation of the material causes significant rise in core body temperature and profuse perspiration. In addition, the front location of the zip imposes additional risk of contamination when the worker undresses the suit. Despite these important shortcomings,

**Table 2 Personal Protective Equipment for High- and Low-risk Patient Areas,
(adopted from the guidelines of the Health Authority, Hong Kong Special
Administration Region[11])**

	High-risk Category	Low-risk Category
Definition	• SARS cohort and screening wards • Fever triage areas • Intensive care unit • Any designated areas for SARS	• All other areas

Mask	• N95 or higher level of protection
	• Fit test if available
		• Surgical mask for
		  routine use
		• N95 for high risk
		  procedures

Eye protection	• Face shield • Goggle for high risk procedures	• Face shield and goggle for high risk procedures
Gown	• Full-length disposable gown	• Optional • Required for high-risk procedures
Gloves	• Latex gloves	• Optional • Required for high-risk procedures

healthcare workers were initially reluctant to part with the Barrier Man. This phenomenon illustrates that fear is a major obstacle to proper implementation of good infection control measures. Good communication and proper dissemination of information are crucial in overcome the emotional distress of the staff in the event of a crisis.

It might be necessary to point out the controversy of whether N95 mask is necessary or simply a surgical mask is sufficient. Both CDC and WHO specifically stated that N95 respirators should be used by healthcare personnel involved in the care of SARS patients.

Regular breaks are essential to relieve stress and to reduce the total exposure to the virus. Extensive nursing procedures for dependent, confused or uncooperative patients could conter high risk of infection to healthcare workers, and therefore should be avoided. All supporting staff should receive proper instructions and supervision on handling of patient's excreta and soiled material. All staff should be reminded not to touch their face and personal protective equipment with contaminated gloves. Hand washing is essential and so is access to clean water. All staff must wash their hands with soap and water before and after contact with SARS patients, after procedures likely to cause contamination as well as after removal gloves or gowns. Alcohol-based handrubs could be used if

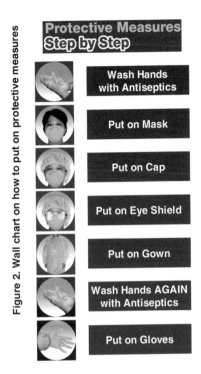

Figure 2. Wall chart on how to put on protective measures

Fig. 2 Wall chart on how to put on protective measures.

there is no obvious organic matter contamination, though hand washing is preferred.

All staff and visitors should put on protective apparels in a designated area. Proper removal of contaminated items is crucial to avoid cross contamination. These procedures should be illustrated by a wall-chart and a dedicated staff member should be present to ensure compliance (Fig. 2). A unit infection control officer should be appointed to reinforce compliance and to carry out spot checks. All staff should be reminded that protective equipment is not meant to be foolproof. Healthcare workers should be allowed to take a shower when they are exposed to respiratory or body secretions, or following aerosol-generating procedures.

CONTROL OF ENVIRONMENTAL FACTORS

Given the prolonged survival of SAR-CoV in the environment, surfaces should be cleaned by staff with proper protection equipment using broad-spectrum disinfectants such as sodium hypochlorite (1 in 50 dilution), or

70% alcohol at least twice daily, or after patients have been vacated. Disposable equipment should be used wherever possible and disposed off properly. Reusable items should be disinfected according to the manufactures' recommendations. Non-essential items should be removed from tabletops or shelves. Disposal plastic bags or lining should be used to contain or cover keyboards, pages, telephones and handsets; these wrappings should be replaced or cleaned twice daily.

Breakthrough transmission occurs in healthcare workers despite use of full protective gear during procedures that produce large amount of aerosols. Hence, nebulizers and noninvasive positive pressure ventilation (e.g. CPAP, BiPAP) should only be used with great caution. For patients with airflow obstruction, the use of metered dose of brochodilator through a spacer device has been shown to be equally effective in relieving bronchospasm compared with the nebulized bronchodilators.[12] For those who develop respiratory failure, BiPAP and CPAP under low pressure may be used before mechanical ventilation is given. It is of paramount importance that these procedures should be performed in an isolation room with negative pressure. If an airborne isolation room is not available, the procedure should be done in a single room with either a high air exchange rate or directional airflow. HEPA filtration units should be used if recirculation of air is unavoidable. Cough producing procedures such as chest physiotherapy, suction, bronchoscopy or gastroscopy should be kept to a minimum and be performed by experienced staff. Personal protection equipment for aerosol-generating procedures must cover the arms and torso, and fully protect the nose, mouth and eyes (goggles and face shields). Higher levels of respiratory protection should be used and they include powered air purifying respirator with loose fitting face pieces or hoods that completely cover the head, neck and portions of shoulders and torso.[13] (Fig. 3).

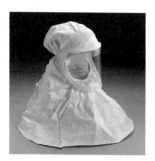

Fig. 3 An example of the powered air purifying respirator.

SURVEILLANCE OF HEALTHCARE WORKERS

Active surveillance for fever and respiratory symptoms is an integral part of infection control measures in view of the high incidence of SARS among healthcare workers. In the early phase of the epidemic, healthcare workers acquired the infection through close and unprotected contact with infected persons. Following the introduction of infection control precautions, breakthrough transmissions still occur sporadically. Monitoring of the staffs well-being is therefore necessary to identify workers who are ill, so that appropriate care and isolation can be given without further delay. Employee absenteeism should be reviewed for any increases that may suggest an emerging illness. A list of staff who have had contact with SARS patients should be maintained. All staff should measure their body temperature at least twice daily.

Workers with unprotected exposure should monitor their body temperature and respiratory symptoms as described previously. They should refrain from going to work if they develop fever or respiratory symptoms; they should stay at home and report to the relevant health service immediately. Their progress should be monitored closely with regular blood tests and chest X-ray. Staff should only return to work 72 hours after resolution of fever or respiratory symptoms and consultation with an occupational health or infection control unit. For those exposed with protection during aerosol-generating procedures and are asymptomatic, they should be quarantined for a 10-day period at home because of the high risk nature of these procedures.

OUTBREAK INVESTIGATION

All cases of transmission of SARS within a hospital should be investigated by a dedicated team. Exposure of staff and other patients to an index case should be established so that at risk subjects can be monitored closely. Any breach in the infection control procedures should be identified and rectified.

Following the outbreaks in hospitals, SARS spread to the community. Studies on transmission dynamics have estimated that each single case of SARS will lead to about three secondary cases in the population during the early phase of the epidemic.[14,15] Contact tracing is essential to identify exposed persons. In Hong Kong, Taiwan, Singapore and Toronto, quarantine of contacts of known SARS patients were carried out to restrict their movements. The quarantine measure is very effective in reducing the spread of SARS among the community and contributes to the breaking of the human chain transmission of SARS.

TRAINING AND IMPLEMENTATION OF INFECTION CONTROL MEASURES

For the health care workers who are not familiar with infection control measures, the procedures of infection control are often deemed to be excessive and unnecessary and hence, compliance is usually poor in the early phase of the outbreak. The poor compliance contributes to the high breakthrough infection rates in the early period of the outbreak. Good communication is required to explain and persuade staff to adhere to these measures. Guidelines and protocols of infection control must be made available to all staff concerned. Educational sessions and demonstrations of practical procedures should be organized and attendance of these training sessions is compulsory. To implement the infection control measures, one member of a unit must be appointed as the infection control officer who has the responsibility to ensure the guidelines are enforced. Audit on the compliance should be carried out regularly. Infection control mechanism should be consolidated to ensure effective implementation of precaution at all workplaces.

CONCLUSION

SARS is a newly emerging disease of this century. Much has been learnt about the virus since its emergence in March 2003, but our understanding of the disease remains very limited. When new information about the disease becomes available, specific measures of infection control should be reviewed accordingly. New guidelines should be promoted to all staff. Although the human chain transmission appears to be broken in July 2003, resurgence of SARS remains a distinct possibility and vigilance must be maintained. One of the characteristics of SARS-CoV is that it will find weaknesses in the healthcare system, no matter how insignificant the fault appeared to be. The success in controlling SARS in hospital demands a high level of collaborations between administrators and healthcare professionals. Effective infection control precautions include onsite assessment of patient characteristics, the environment, clinical activities, staff awareness and compliance. A high level of suspicion, rapid identification and isolation of cases, prompt contact tracing and quarantine are the fundamental steps for the successful control of SARS outbreaks.

REFERENCES

1. Riley S, *et al.* Transmission dynamics of the etiological agent of SARS, in Hong Kong: Impact of public health interventions. *Science* 2003; **300**(5627):1961–6.

2. Centers for Disease Control and Prevention. Use of quarantine to prevent transmission of severe acute respiratory syndrome—Taiwan. *MMWR* 2003;**52**(29):680–3.

3. Lee N, *et al.* A major outbreak of severe acute respiratory syndrome in Hong Kong. *N Engl J Med* 2003;**348**(20):1986–94.

4. Centers for Disease Control and Prevention. Cluster of severe acute respiratory syndrome cases among protected health-care workers—Toronto, Canada. *MMWR* 2003;**52**(19):433–6.

5. Centers for Disease Control and Prevention. From the Centers for Disease Control and Prevention. Severe acute respiratory syndrome—Taiwan. *JAMA* 2003;**289**(22):2930–2.

6. Donnelly CA, *et al.* Epidemiological determinants of spread of causal agent of severe acute respiratory syndrome in Hong Kong. *Lancet* 2003;**361**(9371):1761–6.

7. Tomlinson B and Cockram C. SARS: Experience at Prince of Wales Hospital, Hong Kong. *Lancet* 2003;**361**(9368):1486–7.

8. World Health Organization. First data on stability and resistance of SARS coronavirus compiled by members of WHO laboratory network. 2003, World Health Organization.

9. Seto WH, *et al.* Effectiveness of precautions against droplets and contact in prevention of nosocomial transmission of severe acute respiratory syndrome (SARS). *Lancet* 2003;**361**(9368):1519–20.

10. Centers for Disease Control and Prevention. Updated interim domestic guidelines for triage and disposition of patients who may have severe acute respiratory syndrome (SARS). 2003, Centers for Disease Control and Prevention.

11. Health Authority, Infection control precautions in hospitals, 2003. Health Authority, Hong Kong Special Administration Region, the People's Republic of China: Hong Kong.

12. Raimondi AC, *et al.* Treatment of acute severe asthma with inhaled albuterol delivered via jet nebulizer, metered dose inhaler with spacer, or dry powder. *Chest* 1997;**112**(1):24–8.

13. Centers for Disease Control and Prevention. Interim domestic infection control precautions for aerosol-generating procedures on patients with severe acute respiratory syndrome (SARS), 2003. Centers for Disease Control and Prevention.

14. Riley S, *et al.* Transmission dynamics of the etiological agent of SARS in Hong Kong. Impact of public health interventions. *Science* 2003;**300**:1961–6.

15. Lipsitch M, *et al.* Transmission dynamics and control of severe acute respiratory syndrome. *Science* 2003;**300**(5627):1966–70.

19

Nosocomial Infections

Louis Y Chan, Hong Fung

INTRODUCTION

Nosocomial transmission has been a common feature of the Severe Acute Respiratory Syndrome (SARS) since its emergence. Around the world, many outbreaks had been reported in hospital settings. A patient who traveled from Hong Kong to Vietnam had led to infection of 37 healthcare workers in a hospital in Hanoi.[1] In Singapore, five index cases had transmitted the disease to 90 healthcare workers and in-patients in hospital settings. Despite the rapid accumulation of knowledge of the epidemiology and implementation of infection control measures, nosocomial outbreak still occurred. In mid-April 2003, infection in a single healthcare worker led to SARS infection in more than a hundred staff, patients, and visitors in Taiwan.[2]

Nosocomial transmission of SARS can occur among healthcare workers, patients, and visitors. The secondary attack rate of SARS in hospital seems to be very high. In both Hong Kong and Hanoi, an attack rate of more than 50% has been observed among healthcare workers at the early phase of the outbreak.[3] In Toronto, the attack rate among nurses who worked in the Emergency Department, intensive care unit and coronary care unit, ranged from 10.3% to 60.0%.[4] Many factors may account for the transmission of SARS in hospital settings.

FACTORS LEADING TO NOSOCOMIAL TRANSMISSION OF SARS

Diagnosis and Placement

Achieving the correct diagnosis and appropriate placement is the most crucial but also the most difficult part in the control of nosocomial transmission of SARS. In a SARS screening clinic at the Prince of Wales Hospital, using the WHO criteria (high fever, respiratory symptoms, and history of close contact) for case finding, Rainer *et al.* found a sensitivity of only 26% at presentation. Even chest radiography may not always provide the answer. Pneumonic change on chest radiograph was only presented in 56% of patients at first presentation.[5] Despite the availability of the PCR testing for SARS-CoV, the detection rate in the first week of illness is still far from optimal.[6] Because of the limitations of the clinical criteria and laboratory testing, it is very difficult to be certain about the diagnosis during the early phase of the illness. As a consequence, physicians often need to admit uncertain cases to the hospital. The question is "What is the threshold of admission for suspected SARS cases?"

One may choose to admit patients with the slightest suspicion of SARS to the hospital. The advantage of this approach is that SARS patients will be isolated in the hospital, thereby reducing the risk of transmission of the disease in the community. Epidemiological data suggested that a reduction of duration between symptoms onset and hospitalization contributed to a decrease in the SARS transmission rate in the community.[7] However, there are a number of disadvantages of this approach. Firstly, because of the lack of a large number of isolation/single rooms in most hospitals, patients with suspected SARS may need to be isolated in groups in ward cubicles. This may lead to cross infection among patients. Secondly, the hospital system will rapidly become saturated with a large number of patients with respiratory and febrile symptoms, who normally do not require admission. This will paralyze hospital service for other illnesses. In addition, a heavy workload may contribute to lapses in infection control precautions and lead to SARS infection in healthcare workers.

Degree and Duration of Contact

Close contact is defined by WHO as having cared for, lived with, or had direct contact with respiratory secretions or body fluids of a suspect or probable case of SARS. Current evidences suggested that SARS is mainly transmitted by contact with body fluids and close contact with infected patients. Frequent close contact for a long duration in hospital settings is inevitable. Healthcare workers and relatives often need to nurse patients, especially those who are old and frail and requiring assistance for daily activities. Procedures such as feeding put carers at risk of exposure to patients' oral and respiratory secretions. Since SARS-CoV are also present in urine and feces of SARS patients, healthcare workers are also exposed to high concentrations of virus during handling of patients' urinals and bed pans. In our hospital, we noticed that healthcare workers' infection rate is higher in wards with elderly and dependent patients. This might be related to the heavy nursing required by these patients.

Procedures

Since SARS is mainly transmitted via respiratory droplets, aerosolization of respiratory secretions may potentiate the infectivity of the disease. During the early phase of the outbreak, over 100 healthcare workers, medical students, in-patients, and visitors in a general medical ward were infected with SARS in a matter of a few days.[8] The index patient was admitted seven days after illness onset, and a jet nebulizer was prescribed two days after admission to facilitate mucociliary action and coughing up of sputum. It was noted that in patients who had had contact with the index patient but were discharged before the use of the nebulizer, none of them became infected. On the contrary, half of the patients exposed to the aerosols generated by the jet nebulizer became infected. Therefore, aerosol-generating patient-care procedures pose serious threats to healthcare workers.[9] Through a case control study, a group of investigators also found that the use of high flow oxygen (at 15 L per min) might have contributed to SARS breakthrough infection in two healthcare workers despite adequate personal protective equipment (PPEs) being used.[10] They suggested that high flow oxygen therapy should only be used in isolation rooms.

Endotracheal intubation of SARS patients should be treated as a high risk procedure. This is because airway intubation often causes an awake or a semi-conscious patient to cough. Suctioning of respiratory secretions to clear the airway is often required. Cluster of SARS cases among healthcare workers involved in airway intubation had been reported. In Toronto, six healthcare workers present during the intubation procedure of an index patient contracted SARS, despite the fact that they had adequate PPEs.[9] In Hong Kong, one physician and one nurse who were involved in the intubation of an unsuspected SARS patient became infected and eventually died.

Physical Environment

World Health Organization[11] suggested that SARS patients should be isolated and accommodated as follows, in descending order of preference:

1. negative pressure rooms with the door closed
2. single rooms with attached bathroom facilities
3. cohort placement in an area with an independent air supply, exhaust system and bathroom facilities.

However, it is difficult in most localities to have isolation or single rooms for all probable and suspected SARS in-patients because of the large caseload during the epidemics. (At the peak of the outbreak, there were more than 700 probable SARS cases, and many more suspected cases, in Hong Kong). Therefore, many hospitals have to cohort patients with probable cases of SARS together in designated wards (SARS wards) and patients with suspected SARS in other wards (suspected SARS wards). However, there are a number of limitations to this isolation policy. Firstly, physical spacing in hospital is limited. Beds are located within arm's reach of each other. Toilets and bathrooms are shared among all patients. The scarcity of space and facilities had made prevention of cross infection exceedingly difficult. Suspected SARS patients (who in fact do not have SARS) might get infected by other SARS patients during their stay in the suspected SARS wards. Secondly, the large number of SARS patients in a few designated wards means that the viral load was probably very high and even a minor breach of the protection barrier would put healthcare workers at considerable risk of being infected. Although it is believed that the main route of SARS transmission is respiratory droplets, transmission via other routes such as fomite remains possible. Virology studies have shown that SARS-CoV can survive on dry surfaces for up to three days, signifying the importance of environmental factors in the control of nosocomial transmission of SARS.

Patient Factors

Viral load

Early studies of viral titers in nasopharyngeal aspirates suggest that viral shedding was highest 10 days after the onset of symptoms.[6] Therefore, the infectivity of SARS may be highest around this period. This might explain the frequent occurrence of nosocomial SARS transmission because patients are usually admitted during the period of heavy viral shedding.

Hidden patients

The problem of patients with atypical presentations has been mentioned in previous chapters. These patients became hidden reservoir of infection in the wards of healthcare facilities. Widespread transmissions may occur before identification of these patients. In Singapore, three patients with atypical presentations had resulted in SARS infection in 78 individuals.[12] The problem of hidden SARS patients remains a major challenge in the control of nosocomial SARS transmission.

Superspreader

Epidemiological studies showed that in the majority of patients, SARS is only moderately transmissible, with one case transmitted to three secondary cases in a population that has not yet instituted infection control measures.[13] However, there is a large variation in infectivity among different individuals. In a study of household transmission, it was noticed that only 10% of infected individuals transmitted the disease to their family members. But in those who transmitted the disease to their household members, almost all of their family members were infected.[14] Therefore, some patients appear to be much more infectious than others. The term super-spreading event has been used to describe situations in which a single individual (the super-spreader) has directly infected a large number of other people.[13] A super-spreader has been arbitrary defined as a person who directly infects 10 or more other persons.[12] Super-spreaders have also been described in other diseases such as rubella, laryngeal tuberculosis, and Ebola. We are not sure what constitutes a super-spreading event. It could be viral, host, environmental factors, or indeed a combination of these factors, which greatly enhanced the infectivity of some individuals. In hospital settings, super-spreaders are particularly problematic because patients and staff are in close contact for a long period of time, and this may lead to a large scale point source outbreak. As mentioned above, one of the important factors of SARS transmission is heavy nursing care required by some SARS patients in hospital. Apart from this, some other factors relating to patients might also contribute to nosocomial SARS transmission. For instance, patients often refuse to wear a mask. Patients with dementia are not able to follow instructions, not to mention difficulties with psychiatric patients. Fortunately, we have not had any outbreaks occurring in psychiatric hospitals.

PREVENTION OF SARS NOSOCOMIAL TRANSMISSION

Prevention of transmission in hospitals plays a major role in the control of infection and minimizes the damage caused by SARS to the community. In many localities (such as Hong Kong, Singapore, and Toronto) with major SARS outbreaks, hospitals were the first place where large scale transmissions occurred, before widespread infection in the community. Moreover, hospitalized patients are often old and frail with co-morbidities, hence SARS infection in this group of people carries a much higher mortality than in the general population. In addition, prevention of infection in healthcare workers is of paramount importance to maintain services and staff morale.

DIAGNOSIS AND PLACEMENT

Before a sensitive laboratory test during the early phase of the illness becomes available, it remains difficult to improve the diagnostic accuracy of SARS at presentation. When the diagnosis is uncertain, physicians may also take into account the patients' characteristics in determining whether to admit a patient or not. For young persons with a residential environment suitable for home quarantine, they may be discharged and followed up closely with repeat laboratory and radiographic assessments. It should be clearly conveyed to these patients that the diagnosis is uncertain and they may be infectious. They should refrain from going to work or school, wear surgical masks at home, and avoid close contact with family members. For aged patients (especially those residing in eldercare homes); patients unable to follow instructions (such as psychiatric patients); or those with suboptimal home environment unsuitable for quarantine, it may be better to admit them into a hospital with proper isolation facilities in order to prevent spread in the community. In the hospital, a triage system is required to cohort patient with different indexes of suspicion of having SARS. A model that is adopted by many hospitals in Hong Kong has been published.[15]

Infection in Healthcare Workers

The importance of provision of training in infection control procedures and psychological preparation of healthcare workers before deploying staff to SARS wards cannot be over-emphasized. Simplification and reduction of nursing procedures can help to reduce the duration of contact between staff and patients. The staff-to-patient ratio should be increased in wards with elderly and dependent patients. Movement of staff among different wards should be avoided, as working in an unfamiliar environment and with different teammates often leads to lapses in infection control. Staff should be redeployed as a team instead of members being redeployed from various units on an ad hoc basis. All wards and units should keep a list of working staff with their contact details and time of work. This will facilitate contact tracing in case of any outbreaks.

In order to improve the nursing efficiency, it is not uncommon for many nursing teams to use the "division of labor" strategy. For example, one nurse may measure the blood pressure and body temperature of all the patients in the ward at a designated time. This should now be avoided because healthcare workers will be in close contact with many more patients. Nurses should be assigned a few designated patients and be responsible for all the nursing procedures for these patients. This will minimize the number of staff being exposed to each individual patient and reduce the risk of cross infection.

Cross infection among healthcare workers is possible even outside the ward environment. In order to minimize cross-infection between healthcare workers, several policies have been adopted in hospitals taking care of SARS patients. Staff should avoid unprotected close contact with one another, such as dining together and sharing of eating utensils.

No food or drink is allowed in any place near the wards. Sharing of personal amenities such as pens, mobile phones and stethoscopes should be discouraged. Seats in the cafeteria are placed in one direction so that face-to-face contact is minimized. In some hospitals, glass or plastic shields are installed to reduce droplet transmission.

Physical Environment

Admission of all probable and suspected SARS cases to isolation/single rooms would be the ideal way to prevent cross infection. However, this is difficult to achieve due to resources limitation, especially when the number of patients is large. Therefore, other measures should be sought to optimize the environment. Regular cleansing with disinfectant can effectively reduce the viral load and possibly prevent transmission by fomite. Spacing out of patients in open wards can help to prevent cross infection among them. As the infection is transmitted by droplets and possibly through air, sufficient ventilation should be able to reduce the viral load and hence avoid cross-infection in the hospital. High risk patients should be nursed in rooms with negative pressure. If negative pressure rooms are not available, we have used floor-standing industrial-type HEPA filters to purify the air. These highly efficient filters would clear the air of aerosols down to 0.1–0.4 microns, thus reducing the "carriers" of the virus in air. In China, hospitals open their windows wide and use electric fans to keep air exchange at an adequate level.

Visitors

Visitors should be prohibited in probable and suspected SARS wards. In other areas, the number of visitors and duration of visits should be restricted. All visitors should be checked for their temperature before they enter these areas. Any visitors with fever or respiratory symptoms should be prohibited from entering the premises. Contact information of visitors should be recorded so that they can be contacted in case an outbreak occurs.

Limiting the Spread of Outbreak

Despite all the abovementioned measures, nosocomial SARS transmission might still occur. Early identification of nosocomial transmitted cases, contact tracing and quarantine constitute the most important strategy to halt the transmission chain and reduce the number of infected individuals.

Surveillance for hospital outbreak

Healthcare workers should monitor their temperature twice daily. They should not go to work and inform their managers/supervisors immediately if they develop a fever or respiratory symptoms. The hospital management should closely monitor the sick leave situation of healthcare workers. If a cluster of sick healthcare workers is identified, the possibility of an outbreak should be evaluated. In Taiwan, a laundry worker continued to work in the hospital despite symptoms of fever and diarrhea. He was admitted four days after symptoms onset and SARS was diagnosed two days after admission. Unfortunately, it had resulted in SARS infection in 137 staff, patients, and visitors in the hospital.[16]

The history of visits to a hospital should be explored in all newly diagnosed SARS cases. When a new case of SARS occurred in healthcare workers or patients/visitors, detailed investigations should be performed immediately. The suspected ward(s) or unit(s) where transmission has occurred should be identified. All the patients in the ward should be evaluated to identify possible hidden patient(s). Drastic measures have to be taken in order to prevent further spread within the hospital and to the community. All in-patients who had had close contact with the SARS patient(s) in the hospital should be quarantined. Discharged patients should be quarantined at home.

Healthcare workers who have cared for or otherwise have been exposed to SARS patients while adhering to the recommended infection control precautions need not be put on quarantine, but they should be instructed to be vigilant in case of any fever and respiratory symptoms. However, if the infection control precautions were absent or breached, the concerned healthcare workers should be excluded from duties for 10 days.[17] They should be contacted by occupational health and infection control personnel or their designates regularly over the 10-day period following exposure, to monitor for any development of fever or respiratory symptoms.

Quarantine

The period of quarantine is determined by the incubation period of the disease. The incubation period of SARS is usually 2–7 days, and 10 days is the cutoff used in case definition and quarantine period in most countries. However, clinicians should be aware that the incubation period can be as long as 14 days.[18] and the quarantine period of 10 days is not 100% safe. We encountered a patient who had had close contact with a SARS patient in hospital, and she remained asymptomatic after home quarantine for 10 days. On day 13, she traveled abroad and developed fever upon arrival. SARS was diagnosed and it is believed that she became infected during her hospital stay 13 days ago.[19] Fortunately, she did not lead to any secondary cases of SARS infection.

Analysis of infected healthcare workers

If transmission occurred from patients to healthcare workers despite the use of adequate PPEs, structured investigation should be conducted in order to identify the most likely cause of the transmission, as well as to determine the actions necessary to eliminate it. This includes a detailed face to face interview with the infected staff, interviews with his/her supervisor, and inspection of the work environment. Case control studies (which involve interviews with non-infected staff working in the same environment) might help to identify breaches in infection control measures that have led to the transmission. These investigations should be performed as early as possible to reduce recall bias.

CONCLUSION

In many countries where the SARS outbreak had occurred, hospitals were the first place where large scale transmission took place. This is largely due to the lack of knowledge of and alertness to the disease. With the increasing understanding of SARS and the heightened level of vigilance, we should be more equipped to prevent further hospital outbreak next round when SARS returns.

REFERENCES

1. Centers for Disease Control and Prevention. Updated: Outbreak of Severe Acute Respiratory Syndrome — Worldwide, *MMWR Morb Mortal Wkly Rep* 2003;**52**:241–248.

2. Centers for Disease Control and Prevention. Updated: Severe Acute Respiratory Syndrome — United States, *MMWR Morb Mortal Wkly Rep* 2003;**52**:466–468.

3. Centers for Disease Control and Prevention. Outbreak of Severe Acute Respiratory Syndrome — Worldwide, *MMWR Morb Mortal Wkly Rep* 2003;**52**:226–228.

4. Monali Varia, Samantha Wilson, Shelly Sarwal, Varia M, Wilson S, Sarwal S, *et al.* Investigation of a nosocomial outbreak of severe acute respiratory syndrome (SARS) in Toronto, Canada, *CMAJ* 2003;**169**: 285–92.

5. Rainer TH, Cameron PA, Smit D, *et al.* Evaluation of WHO criteria for identifying patients with severe acute respiratory syndrome out of hospital: Prospective observational study, *BMJ* 2003;**326**:1354–8.

6. Peiris JS, Chu CM, Cheng VC, *et al.* HKU/UCH SARS Study Group. Clinical progression and viral load in a community outbreak of coronavirus-associated SARS pneumonia: A prospective study, *Lancet* 2003;**361**:1767–72.

7. Riley S, Fraser C, Donnelly CA, *et al.* Transmission dynamics of the etiological agent of SARS in Hong Kong: Impact of public health interventions, *Science* 2003;**300**:1961–6.

8. Lee N, Hui D, Wu A, *et al.* A major outbreak of severe acute respiratory syndrome in Hong Kong, *N Engl J Med* 2003;**348**:1986–94.

9. Centers for Disease Control and Prevention. Cluster of Severe Acute Respiratory Syndrome cases among protected health-care workers — Toronto, Canada, *MMWR Morb Mortal Wkly Rep* 2003;**52**: 433–436.

10. Seto WH. Epidemiology update on SARS situation in Queen Mary Hospital 14/05/03.

11. World Health Organization. Hospital Infection Control Guidance for Severe Acute Respiratory Syndrome (SARS). http://www.who.int/csr/sars/infectioncontrol/en/.

12. Centers for Disease Control and Prevention. Severe Acute Respiratory Syndrome — Singapore, *MMWR Morb Mortal Wkly Rep* 2003;**52**:405–411.

13. Lipsitch M, Cohen T, Cooper B, *et al.* Transmission dynamics and control of severe acute respiratory syndrome, *Science* 2003;**300**(5627): 1966–70.

14. Chan LY, JTH Wong, PKT Li, *et al.* Risk of transmission of Severe Acute Respiratory Syndrome to household contacts from infected health care workers and patients, *Am J Med* (in press).

15. Ho W. Guideline on management of severe acute respiratory syndrome (SARS), *Lancet* 2003;**361**:1313–5.

16. Centers for Disease Control and Prevention. Severe acute respiratory syndrome–Taiwan, *MMWR Morb Mortal Wkly Rep* 2003;**52**:461–6.

17. Centers for Disease Control and Prevention. Interim Domestic Guidance for Management of Exposures to Severe Acute Respiratory Syndrome (SARS) for Health-Care Settings. http://www.cdc.gov/ncidod/sars/exposureguidance.htm.

18. Donnelly CA, Ghani AC, Leung GM, *et al.* Epidemiological determinants of spread of causal agent of severe acute respiratory syndrome in Hong Kong, *Lancet* 2003;**361**:1761–6.

19. Department of Health press release. DH notified of a SARS case by Guangdong. http://www.info.gov.hk/gia/general/200306/25/0625290.htm.

20

Will the SARS Epidemic Recur?

Joseph JY Sung

SARS is the first severe and readily transmissible disease that emerged in the 21st century. It has a unique capacity of spreading quickly in hospitals and clinics, affecting thousands of healthcare workers in a short period of time. The escalation of international air travel in the recent decades has also aided the rapid spread of infection across the continents. In March 2003, one infected tourist from China checked into a hotel in Hong Kong and spread the infection to eight countries within two weeks. By July 2003, 32 countries were involved and 8439 patients were infected around the world. Like many viral infections of the respiratory system, SARS seems to have a seasonality. Although WHO has announced that the initial crisis is over, we should not be complacent. SARS might return in the winter.

This prediction is based on three reasons. First, despite much effort contributed by virologists and molecular biologists, we are still not sure of the source of the infection. Early reports suggested that SARS-CoV resembled the bovine coronavirus or mouse hepatitis virus. Yet, after the sequence of the whole viral genome was completed, it became clear that the SARS-CoV is a distinctly new pathogenic strain that does not arise from a simple recombination of known existing strains. But, we are still not sure

251

where it comes from. Recently, SARS-CoV-like viruses have been isolated from the Himalayan palm civets in a live animal market in Guangdong province of southern China. In addition to palm civets, a similar virus has also been detected in other animals, including a raccoon dog and in retailers working in the animal market. However, this animal strains of SARS-CoV is not identical to that of the human SARS-CoV. All the animal isolates retain a 29-nucleotide sequence which is not found in the human isolates. We cannot be certain that the SARS-CoV is a mutated strain of the animal CoV. Yet, the detection of SARS-CoV-like viruses in small wild mammals in animal markets suggests that a route of inter-species transmission is possible. Not until we can find the source of infection and its natural reservoir, we eliminate the possibility of a return of the infection.

Second, serological studies have revealed that asymptomatic or sub-clinical infection of SARS-CoV is uncommon. We examined 674 healthcare workers at the Prince of Wales Hospital, where the first hospital outbreak occurred in Hong Kong; among them 43% had direct contact with SARS patients. None of them had IgG antibody to SARS-CoV. Another study was conducted in Hong Kong in which donation of serum was solicited from healthcare workers in the primary care sector. Hundreds of serum samples were tested. Less than 5% of samples were positive for IgG SARS-CoV. Similar studies conducted in China confirmed that asymptomatic carriers are few. This implies that immunity to SARS-CoV in the community will develop slowly. Should SARS return, it is likely that another endemic will occur. Based on observations in the last global endemic, hospitals and clinics are the most likely sites of future outbreaks.

Third, although RNA viruses are known to mutate more readily than DNA viruses, genomic studies of SARS-CoV, including strains isolated from Singapore, Hong Kong, Guangdong and Beijing showed a remarkable genetic conservation of the virus since the outbreak first started in November 2002. Unlike most other infectious agents transmitted by direct person-to-person contact, the SARS-CoV is unlikely to mutate to a benign infection and attenuated symptoms. Without herd immunity and attenuation of the virus, when the next epidemic comes, one would still expect to have large-scale outbreaks with severe symptoms.

At the time of writing of this chapter, there is a confirmed case of SARS reported in a virology laboratory in Singapore. A man was hospitalized for fever in Singapore with preliminary test positive for the SARS coronavirus. The symptoms and radiographic changes were compatible with SARS and PCR subsequently confirmed that he had been infected with SARS-CoV. The patient had no history of travel nor any contact with SARS patients. The most likely source of infection was through handling of specimens in the laboratory at the National University Hospital of Singapore. This is the first reported case of a laboratory infection albeit one that involved Level 3 laboratory. He was promptly isolated and soon recovered from the illness. No further outbreak was documented.

What can we do to prepare for a return of SARS? It would be a while before a vaccine can be developed, if it could ever be developed. We should continue to search for the source of the virus and study the mode of transmission of the disease. We should maintain a high level of vigilance of the infection. When we see suspected cases, we should implement isolation, and quarantine and cohorting measures. Developing a rapid diagnostic test, probably PCR-based, which can differentiate SARS from other atypical pneumonia at an earliest possible stage of the disease, would be instrumental in applying these measures successfully.

The following policy should be adopted in countries which are likely to be affected by SARS.

1. Surveillance. Areas with a high risk of outbreak of SARS should keep a high level of alert and continuous surveillance should be adopted. Healthcare workers with fever and symptoms of flu should report promptly to their supervisor and the institution. Daily monitoring of temperature before work should be considered. The other high risk areas would be elderly care as well as homes schools. Vigilance should be maintained in these settings.

2. Education. The public should be well informed about the science of SARS as well as the public health policy aimed at preventing outbreaks. They should understand the importance of personal hygiene as well as environmental sanitation. Educating the public is the most important tool to ensure compliance with public health measures and avoidance of unnecessary phobia.

3. Precautions of droplet infection. Although there could be various ways of transmission SARS, droplet infection is still the most likely route of transmission. During the last endemic, when governments implement the policy of mask-wearing in different countries, the SARS outbreak in the community was stopped. Mask wearing is a small price to pay if there is evidence of an outbreak of SARS in the future.

4. Networking with International Communities. In the last endemic of SARS, containment of the infection was achieved through the efforts of the WHO and CDC, as well as the efforts of national health authorities. It is important to maintain, and promote, networking between these bodies so that information would be communicated without delay. Case reporting should be done expeditiously and outbreaks in local cities should be promptly reported so that the international communities can react accordingly. In this era of electronic communication, messages can be related almost at real time.

5. Prophylaxis and prompt treatment for influenza. Since the symptoms of SARS cannot be differentiated from those of influenza, and the two infections could be recurring at around the same time. Vaccination of high risk individuals (e.g. elderly patients with comorbid illnesses) with influenza vaccine may reduce the confusion of diagnosis and help to control and isolate real cases of SARS.

REFERENCES

1. Marra MA, Jones SJM, Astell CR *et al.* The genome sequence of the SARS-associated coronavirus. Published online May 1, 2003. http://www.sciencemag.org/cgi/rapidpdf/1085953v1.pdf.

2. Chan PKS, Ip M, Ng KC, *et al.* Sero-prevalence of severe acute respiratory syndrome (SARS)-associated coronavirus infection among healthcare workers after a major outbreak of SARS in a regional hospital. *Emerging Infect Dis* (in press).

3. Ruan Y, Wei CL, Ee LA, *et al.* Comparative full-length genome sequence analysis of 14 SARS coronavirus isolates and common mutations associated with putative origins of infection. *Lancet* 2003; **361**:1779–1785.

4. Guan Y, Zheng BJ, He YQ, *et al.* Isolation and characterization of virus related to SARS coronavirus from animals in the southern China. *Sciencexpress* 2003.

Index